AF745558

Cancer Immunotherapy and Biological Cancer Treatments

Edited by Hilal Arnouk

Published in London, United Kingdom

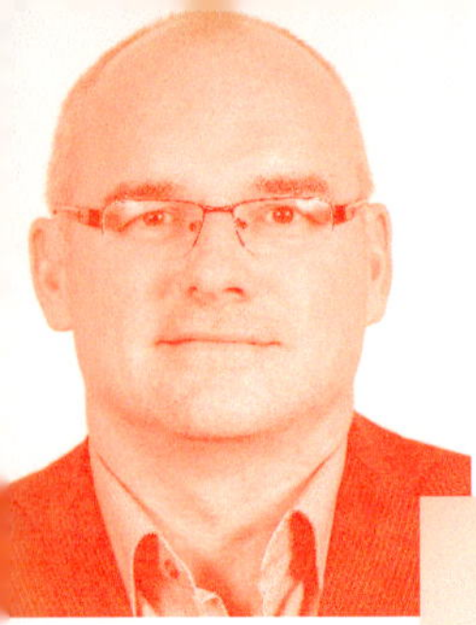
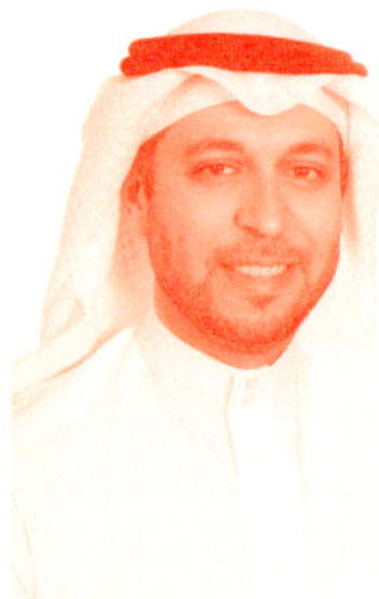
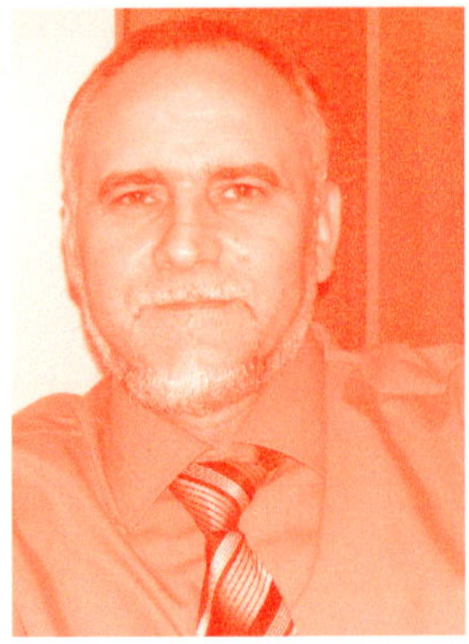
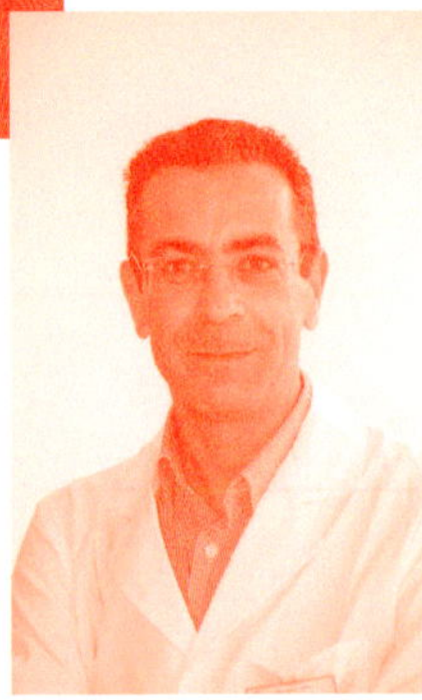
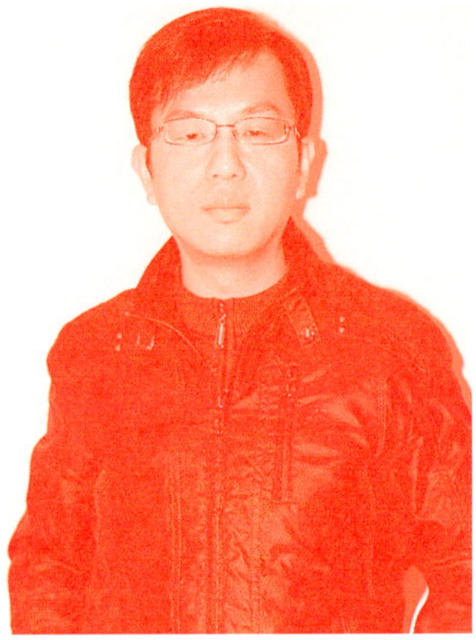
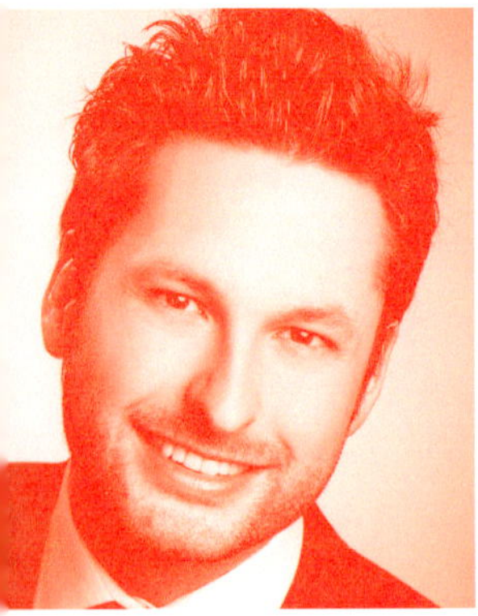
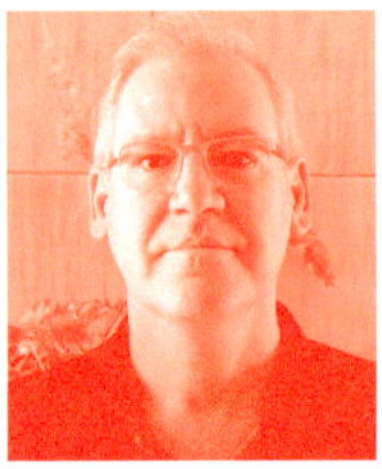

IntechOpen

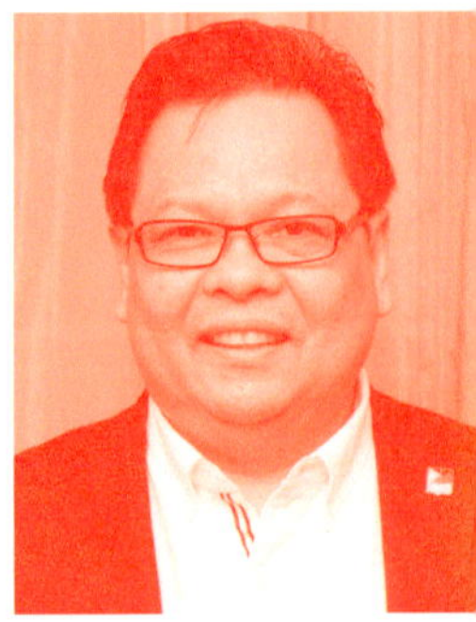
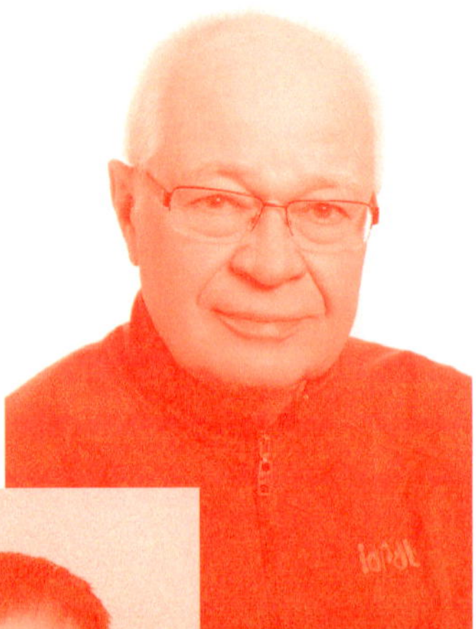
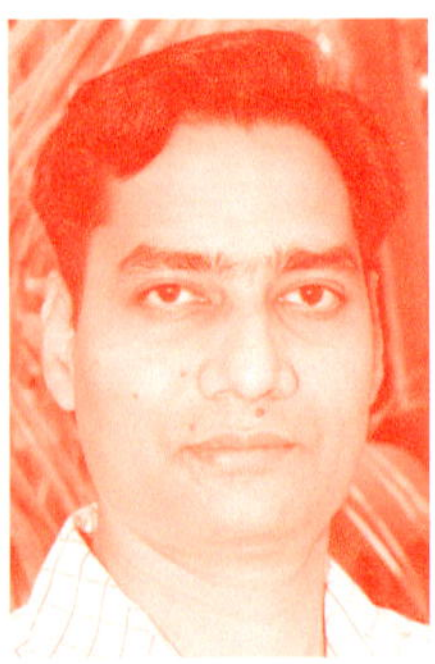
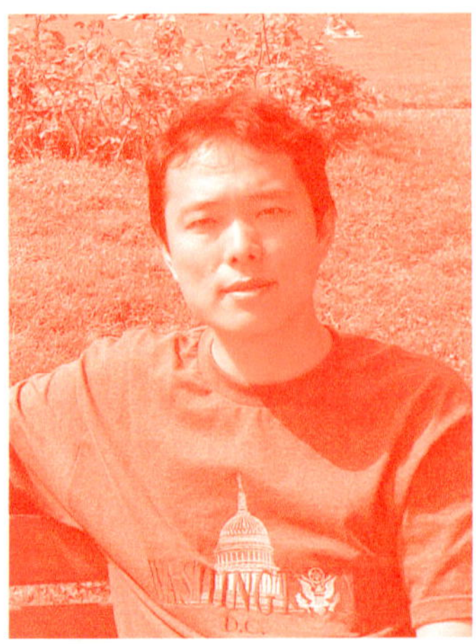
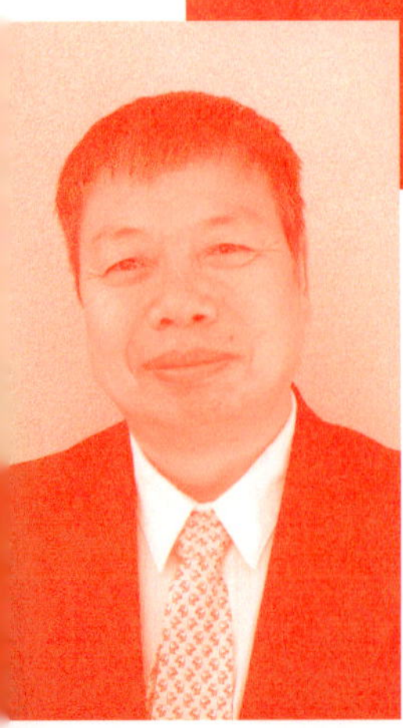
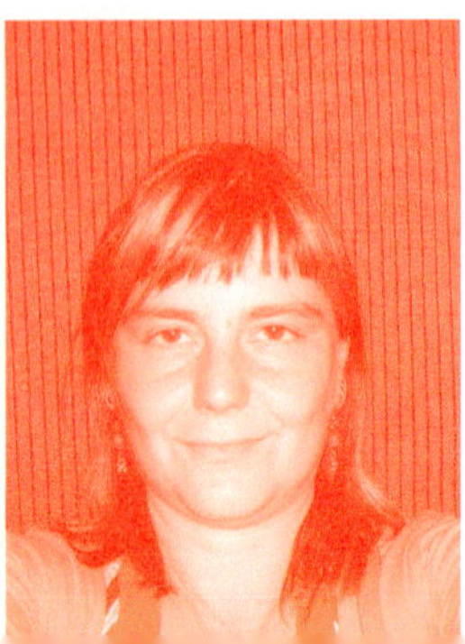

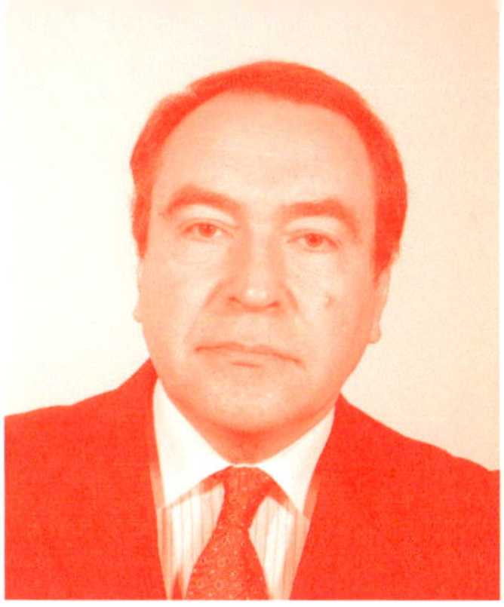
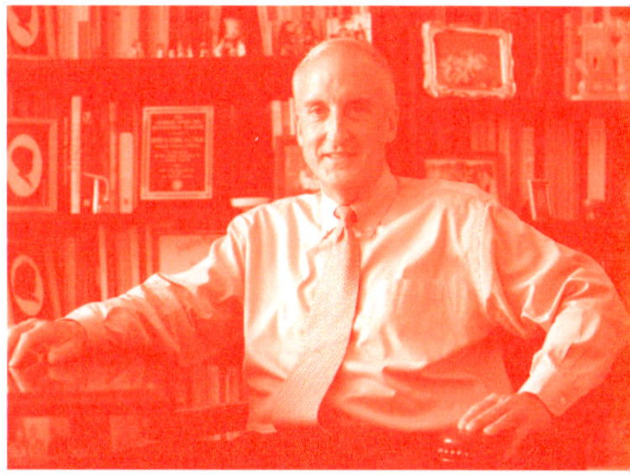
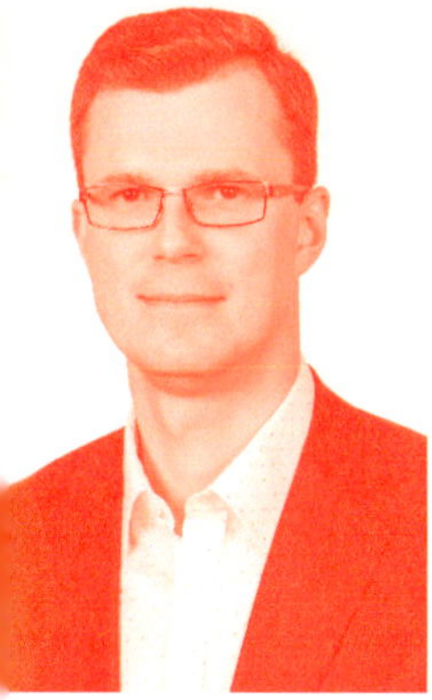
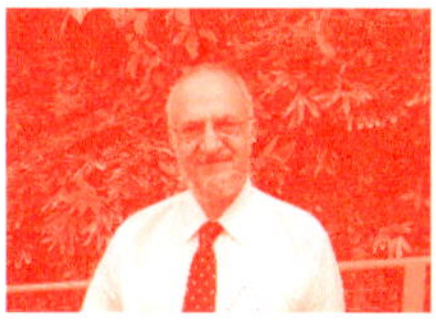
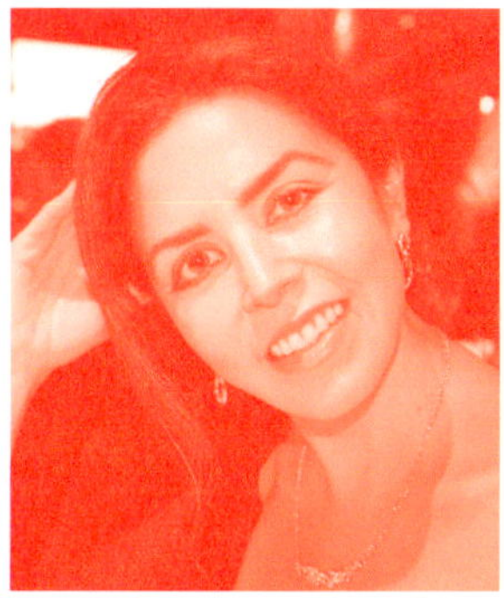

Supporting open minds since 2005

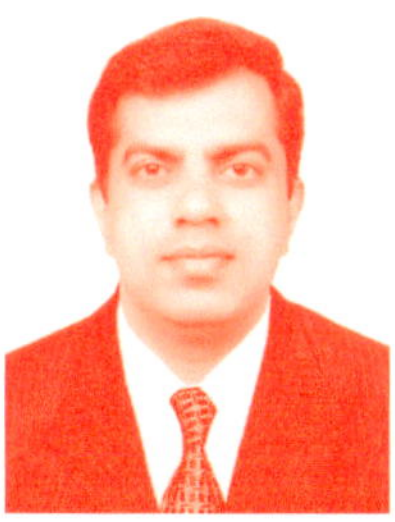
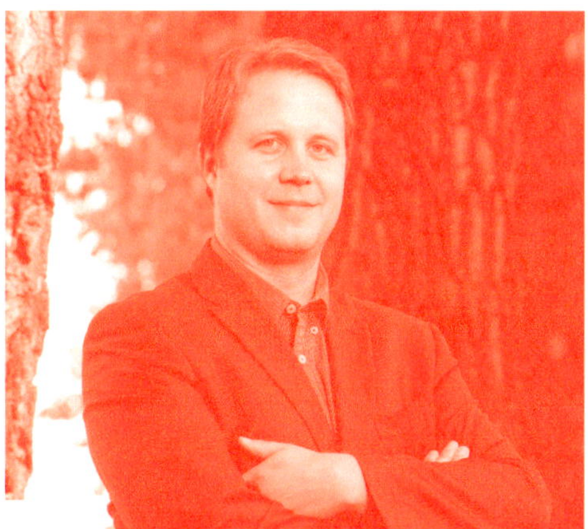
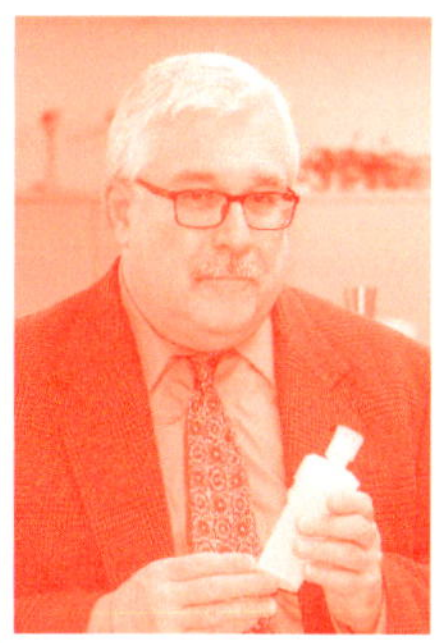
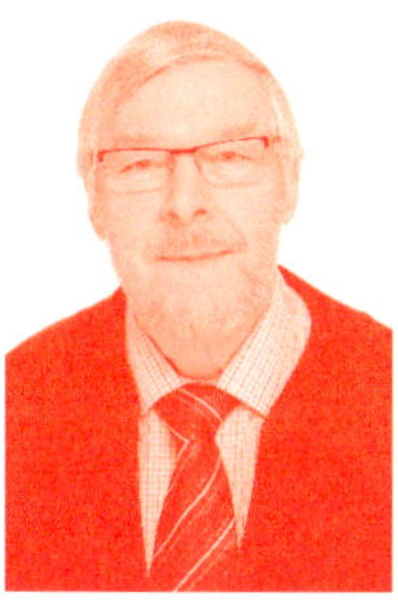
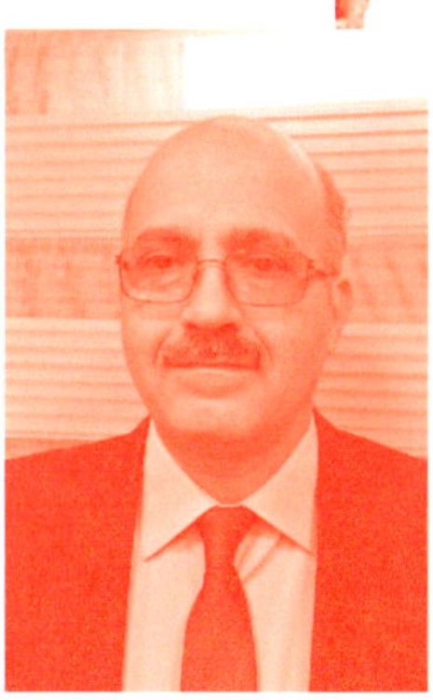
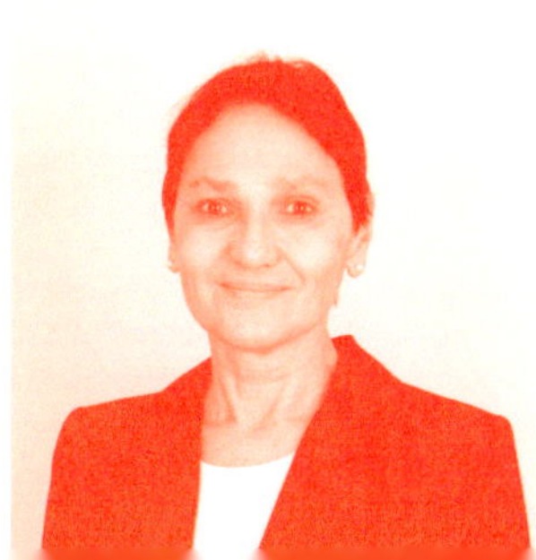
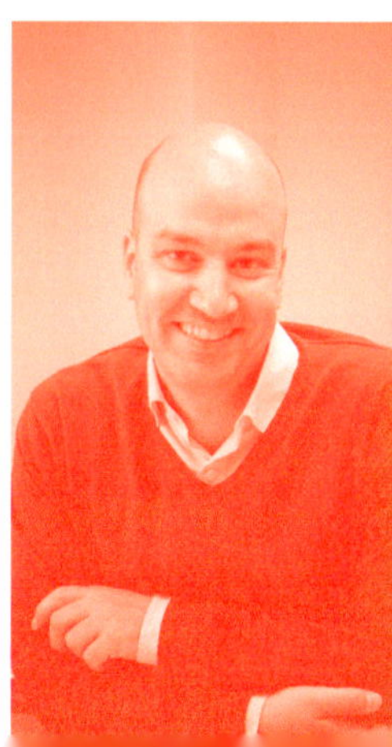

Cancer Immunotherapy and Biological Cancer Treatments
http://dx.doi.org/10.5772/intechopen.77856
Edited by Hilal Arnouk

Contributors
Cristina Pantaleone, Thomas Kieber-Emmons, Anastas Pashov, Suwit Chaisri, Chanvit Leelayuwat, Xiaoming Qi, Yuan Shan, Dongxia Feng, Jason H. Huang, Carmen Murias, Hendrik-Tobias Arkenau, Anna Patrikidou, Valerie Dutoit, Hilal Arnouk, Sana Moqeet

© The Editor(s) and the Author(s) 2019
The rights of the editor(s) and the author(s) have been asserted in accordance with the Copyright, Designs and Patents Act 1988. All rights to the book as a whole are reserved by INTECHOPEN LIMITED. The book as a whole (compilation) cannot be reproduced, distributed or used for commercial or non-commercial purposes without INTECHOPEN LIMITED's written permission. Enquiries concerning the use of the book should be directed to INTECHOPEN LIMITED rights and permissions department (permissions@intechopen.com).
Violations are liable to prosecution under the governing Copyright Law.

Individual chapters of this publication are distributed under the terms of the Creative Commons Attribution 3.0 Unported License which permits commercial use, distribution and reproduction of the individual chapters, provided the original author(s) and source publication are appropriately acknowledged. If so indicated, certain images may not be included under the Creative Commons license. In such cases users will need to obtain permission from the license holder to reproduce the material. More details and guidelines concerning content reuse and adaptation can be found at http://www.intechopen.com/copyright-policy.html.

Notice
Statements and opinions expressed in the chapters are these of the individual contributors and not necessarily those of the editors or publisher. No responsibility is accepted for the accuracy of information contained in the published chapters. The publisher assumes no responsibility for any damage or injury to persons or property arising out of the use of any materials, instructions, methods or ideas contained in the book.

First published in London, United Kingdom, 2019 by IntechOpen
IntechOpen is the global imprint of INTECHOPEN LIMITED, registered in England and Wales, registration number: 11086078, 7th floor, 10 Lower Thames Street, London, EC3R 6AF, United Kingdom
Printed in Croatia

British Library Cataloguing-in-Publication Data
A catalogue record for this book is available from the British Library

Additional hard and PDF copies can be obtained from orders@intechopen.com

Cancer Immunotherapy and Biological Cancer Treatments
Edited by Hilal Arnouk
p. cm.
Print ISBN 978-1-78984-862-5
Online ISBN 978-1-78984-863-2
eBook (PDF) ISBN 978-1-78984-366-8

For EU product safety concerns:
IN TECH d.o.o., Prolaz Marije Krucifikse Kozulić 3, 51000 Rijeka, Croatia, info@intechopen.com or visit our website at intechopen.com.

We are IntechOpen, the world's leading publisher of Open Access books

Built by scientists, for scientists

4,400+
Open access books available

117,000+
International authors and editors

130M+
Downloads

151
Countries delivered to

Our authors are among the
Top 1%
most cited scientists

12.2%
Contributors from top 500 universities

WEB OF SCIENCE™

Selection of our books indexed in the Book Citation Index
in Web of Science™ Core Collection (BKCI)

Interested in publishing with us?
Contact book.department@intechopen.com

Numbers displayed above are based on latest data collected.
For more information visit www.intechopen.com

Meet the editor

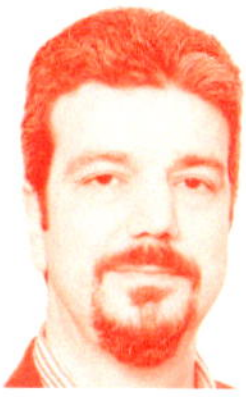

Hilal Arnouk, MD, PhD is an Assistant Professor at the Department of Pathology at Midwestern University. Dr. Arnouk has received his education and post-doctorate training at Roswell Park Cancer Institute, the State University of New York at Buffalo, the Medical College of Georgia and the University of Alabama at Birmingham. He has directed research studies in academia and biotech industry settings. His major areas of expertise include Cancer Immunotherapy, Biomarker Discovery and Precision Medicine. Additionally, Dr. Arnouk enjoys being an educator and mentor for professional students in the medical and biomedical sciences.

Contents

Preface

"To succeed, jump as quickly at opportunities as you do at conclusions."

Benjamin Franklin

In recent years, cancer immunotherapy has emerged as a leading way to combat several different types of cancer. Although the beginnings of cancer immunotherapy date back to the nineteenth century and the experiments of William Coley, recent scientific breakthroughs have allowed medical treatments resulting in increased survival rates of cancer patients. Cancer immunotherapy utilizes different tools, including tumor antigens, cancer vaccines, adoptive cellular immunotherapy, natural killer cell therapy, chimeric antigen receptor T-cell (CAR-T cell) therapy, antibody-based therapy, and immune checkpoint inhibitors. Innovative biological treatments are currently being developed to target malignant tumor cells and to bypass the tumor evasion of the immune system. Notably, CAR-T cell therapy and immune checkpoint inhibitors have made waves of progress in the medical and scientific societies. Other therapies such as cancer vaccines remain revolutionary and have been accepted as forms of treatments for certain types of cancer, including advanced stage prostate cancer. However, challenges remain on how the research and medical communities will be able to efficiently harness the potential of these therapies with minimal side effects. The hope remains that the advancements in the field will allow for greater survival rates and better quality of life for patients inflicted with cancer.

I would like to thank all those who helped with this publication, especially Ms. Dolores Kuzelj. Finally, I dedicate this book to my family, my colleagues, and my mentors and mentees throughout my career.

Hilal Arnouk, MD, PhD
Department of Pathology,
College of Graduate Studies,
Chicago College of Osteopathic Medicine,
College of Dental Medicine-Illinois,
Chicago College of Optometry,
Midwestern University,
Downers Grove, Illinois, United States

Chapter 1

Introductory Chapter: Are We There Yet? The Long and Winding Road to Cancer Immunotherapy

Hilal Arnouk and Sana Moqeet

1. History of cancer immunotherapy

Cancer immunotherapy has become an innovative approach that both pushes the medical and scientific community to better understand our own immune system and charts a new frontier in the fight against one of the leading killers in the world, cancer. The advent of this line of work dates back to the discovery of vaccine. Luminary scientists in the nineteenth century such as Joseph Lister, Louis Pasteur, Robert Koch, and most notably William Coley have allowed for a better understanding of the immune responses and the establishment of vaccines, including vaccines directed against malignant tumors [1–4].

While the basic concept of using immunotherapy to combat cancer was practiced in the scientific community, specifically by Coley, scientists Thomas and Burney were the first to propose the theory of cancer immunosurveillance in 1957. The premise behind their theory was that lymphocytes, an integral part of the immune system, have the capability to eliminate the mutated cancerous cells throughout the human body [5–8]. However, due to a lack of scientific proof-of-concept and the inability to culture the lymphocytes ex vivo for extended periods of time, the next development did not occur until a few decades later. From the 1970s onward, the scientific community has discovered the utility of several different immune therapies to treat cancer including interferon alpha (IFN-α) [9], the T cell growth factor interleukin 2 (IL-2), monoclonal antibodies targeting tumor-associated antigens, and the first FDA-approved cell-based cancer vaccine developed for patients with advanced prostate cancer in 2010 (**Figure 1**).

This chapter will give a brief overview of few of these therapies that scientists and physicians are currently utilizing in the fight against cancer.

2. Tumor antigens

Tumor cells are distinguished from normal cells in a tissue by the presence of unique proteins known as tumor antigens. They can be further divided into two broad categories, tumor-associated antigens and tumor-specific antigens.

Tumor-associated antigens can arise from oncofetal genes that become aberrantly expressed in malignant cells, such as alpha-fetoprotein (AFP) in liver cancer and the melanoma-specific antigens of the MAGE family [10], or from cancer-testis antigens that are expressed normally in the germ cells and become activated in cancers, such as the New York esophageal squamous cell carcinoma 1 (NY-ESO-1) antigen [11]. Tumor-associated antigens also include tissue

IntechOpen

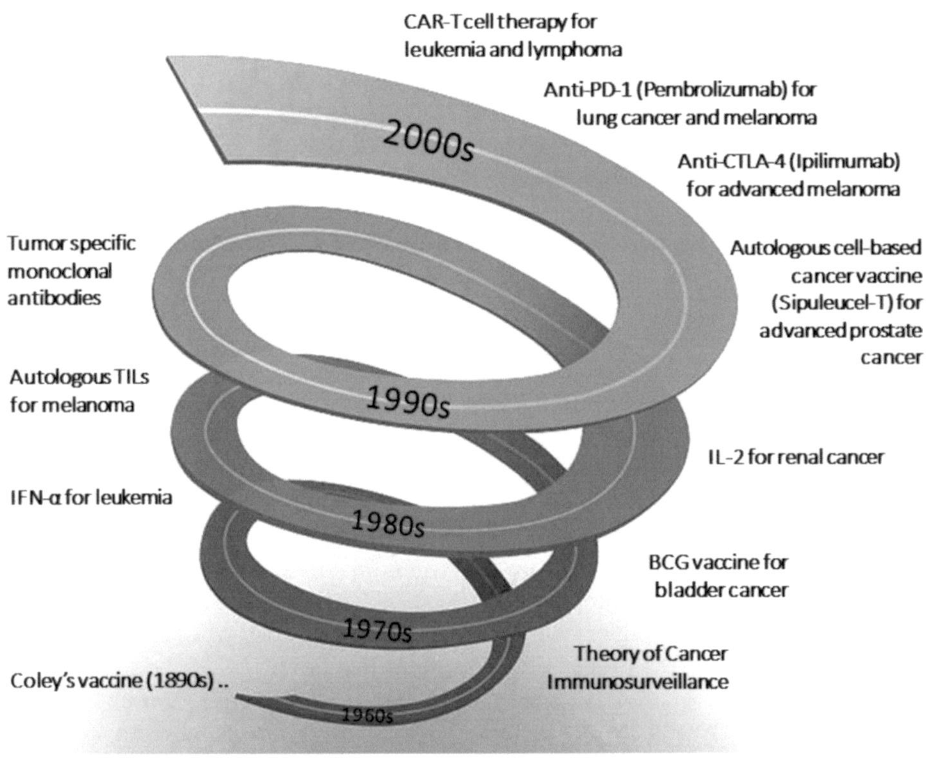

Figure 1.
Key events in the history of cancer immunotherapy.

differentiation antigens, such as tyrosinase in melanoma [12], and viral antigens in a number of malignancies where viral oncogenesis is implicated, such as HPV E6 and E7 oncoproteins in HPV-associated cervical cancers [13]. On the other hand, tumor-specific antigens are usually the products of mutated oncogenes or tumor suppressor genes, such as *ras* and *p53*.

3. Cancer vaccines

While it is well established that vaccines are a way to stimulate the immune system against infectious agents, the concept of harnessing the power of a vaccine to eliminate cancers remains revolutionary. Cancer vaccines work through inducing a specific antitumor T cell response.

Cancer vaccines are divided into prophylactic and therapeutic vaccines. For instance, a prophylactic vaccine against human papillomavirus (HPV) can prevent several cancer types caused by virus, such as cervical cancer and some cancers of the oropharynx [14, 15], and hepatitis B virus (HBV) vaccine provides protection against liver cancers initiated by the hepatitis B virus [16]. Alternatively, therapeutic cancer vaccines trigger an immune response against an existing tumor by inducing T cell response within the tumor microenvironment. Various formats have been developed for therapeutic cancer vaccines, including peptide fragments and full-length tumor antigens, vectors for genetically encoded tumor antigens, whole tumor cell contents, and autologous dendritic cell (DC) vaccines. Most notably, Sipuleucel-T (Provenge) was the first FDA-approved cell-based cancer vaccine developed for patients with hormone-refractory prostate cancer and has shown to prolong the life of affected patients by several months [17, 18].

Since most tumor-associated antigens are not highly immunogenic on their own, an immune adjuvant is typically added to vaccine formulas. Examples of vaccine adjuvants include recombinant granulocyte-macrophage colony-stimulating factor (GM-CSF) and heat shock proteins [19–21].

4. Adoptive cellular immunotherapy

Adoptive cellular immunotherapy (ACT) is the process of transferring effector immune cells, such as T lymphocytes, to cancer patients, including modifying and expanding these immune cells ex vivo to target specific cancer cells [22, 23]. The transferred immune cells can have autologous or allogeneic origin. Two major approaches have been utilized for adoptive cellular immunotherapy, tumor-infiltrating lymphocytes (TILs) and chimeric antigen receptor-modified T cell (CAR-T) therapy.

4.1 Tumor-infiltrating lymphocytes (TILs)

A tumor-infiltrating lymphocyte is an immune cell that has moved into a tumor in the attempt to destroy the cancer. In this therapy, TILs are extracted from tumor tissue biopsies and cultured in vitro with IL-2 to expand the tumor-reactive clones. Once activated, lymphocytes are infused back into the patient [24].

4.2 Chimeric antigen receptor-modified T cell (CAR-T) therapy

Chimeric antigen receptor-modified T cell (CAR-T) therapy has emerged as a successful method in the fight against cancer, especially B cell hematologic malignancies [25]. This success lies within the chimeric antigen receptors (CAR) composed of single-chain variable fragment (scFv) and the costimulatory signaling molecules that can stimulate T cells and allow for direct antigen binding and activation, bypassing the requirement for antigen presentation by antigen-presenting cells (APCs).

CAR-T cell therapy has been especially effective against certain types of lymphoma and leukemia, such as refractory B cell lymphoma and acute lymphoblastic leukemia (ALL) [26, 27]. CAR-T cell therapy is a multistep process. First, patients are evaluated to determine if CAR-T cell therapy is an appropriate treatment. Second, T cells are isolated from blood. The patient's T cells are then taken into the laboratory to be genetically modified to express the chimeric antigen receptors (CARs) on their surfaces. As discussed above, these essential receptors allow for the modified T cells to recognize tumor antigens. Finally, the CAR-T cells are infused back into the patient, and a recovery period of 2–3 months is expected [28].

Overall, CAR-T cell therapy has become a leading area of continued growth and research in the field of cancer immunotherapy. It has had much success in both preclinical and clinical applications, and the next steps involve harnessing the power of modified T cells to aid in eliminating solid tumors including aggressive cancers, such as sarcomas.

4.3 NK cell therapy

Natural killer (NK) cells are large granular lymphocytes that can destroy cells organically, without the requirement for priming first. One of the major hypotheses related to NK cells is the "missing self" hypothesis, which states that NK cells have the ability to destroy cells that do not display major histocompatibility complex

(MHC) class I molecules [29]. Given the extraordinary functions of NK cells in recognizing and destroying altered cells, NK cell-based therapies have become a wide area of research for diseases like cancer. One such targeted therapy is the use of NK alloreactivity, specifically in acute leukemia and other types of hematologic cancers. MHC class I inhibitory receptors, specifically killer immunoglobulin-like receptors (KIRs), have been utilized to exert NK cell alloreactivities as a way to combat leukemic cells [30].

5. Antibody-based treatments

Antibodies are arguably one of the most important aspects of the human immune system. They serve to bind to antigens and allow for flagging of cells with specific antigens for eradication. An antitumor monoclonal antibody is a genetically engineered immunoglobulin that is produced to recognize a specific tumor antigen on the surface of a cancer cell [31].

Monoclonal antibodies work in a multitude of ways including flagging cancer cells, blocking growth of cells, blocking immune inhibitors, directly attacking cancer cells, and bridging cancer and immune cells [32]. Monoclonal antibodies come in two different varieties, naked and conjugated. Naked monoclonal antibodies work individually and can attach themselves to antigens on cancer cells. For instance, trastuzumab (Herceptin) can bind to HER2 oncogene/tumor antigen that is overexpressed in a subset of breast cancers, which blocks the growth and proliferation of the malignant cells [33]. Conjugated monoclonal antibodies work by carrying a radioactive or cytotoxic drug into proximity to the tumor cells, thus killing these malignant cells [34, 35]. As with other cancer immunotherapies, antibody-based treatments carry the risk of adverse side effects that include fever, weakness, nausea, and rashes.

6. Immune checkpoint inhibitors

Immune checkpoint inhibitors are inhibitory molecules on immune cells that prevent the immune system from attacking the organism's own tissues. Two of the identified immune checkpoints are programmed cell death-1 (PD-1) and cytotoxic T lymphocyte-associated protein 4 (CTLA-4) [36].

Interaction of PD-1 and its ligand PDL-1 leads to T lymphocytes' dysfunction and exhaustion. PDL-1 is shown to be highly expressed on cancer cells [37]. Consequently, the blockage of PD-1 and PDL-1 interactions using immune checkpoint inhibitors allows tumor-specific T lymphocytes to exert their function by recognizing and destroying cancer cells. Nivolumab and pembrolizumab are monoclonal antibodies that function as PD-1 blockers and are being currently being used to treat patients with advanced melanoma and non-small cell lung cancer [38, 39]. Similarly, CTLA-4 inhibits T cell activation. Thus, CTLA-4 blockage with inhibitors, such as ipilimumab, enhances the immune responses against malignant tumors such as melanoma [40].

It is important to note, however, that the use of immune checkpoint inhibitors in cancer immunotherapy is frequently followed by inflammatory and autoimmune side effects that include endocrine effects, rash, and hepatitis [41, 42].

In conclusion, cancer immunotherapy remains a field that has tremendously changed our understanding of how to best treat cancers. While advancements have been made, there are many more discoveries to be made as the field of tumor immunology is growing exponentially.

Author details

Hilal Arnouk[1]* and Sana Moqeet[2]

1 Department of Pathology, College of Graduate Studies, Chicago College of Osteopathic Medicine, College of Dental Medicine-Illinois, Chicago College of Optometry, Midwestern University, Illinois, United States

2 Chicago College of Osteopathic Medicine, Midwestern University, Illinois, United States

*Address all correspondence to: harnou@midwestern.edu

IntechOpen

© 2019 The Author(s). Licensee IntechOpen. This chapter is distributed under the terms of the Creative Commons Attribution License (http://creativecommons.org/licenses/by/3.0), which permits unrestricted use, distribution, and reproduction in any medium, provided the original work is properly cited.

References

[1] Gradmann C. A matter of methods: The historicity of Koch's postulates 1840-2000. Medizinhistorisches Journal. 2008;**43**:121-148

[2] Herr HW. Ignorance is bliss: The Listerian revolution and education of American surgeons. The Journal of Urology. 2007;**177**:457-460

[3] Ullmann A. Pasteur-Koch: Distinctive ways of thinking about infectious diseases. Microbe. 2007;**2**:383-387

[4] Coley WB. II. Contribution to the knowledge of sarcoma. Annals of Surgery. 1891;**14**(3):199-220

[5] Thomas L. Discussion of cellular and humoral aspects of hypersensitive states. In: Lawrence HS, editor. New York: Hoeber-Harper; 1959

[6] Burnet FM. Cancer A biological approach. 1. The process of control. British Medical Journal. 1957;**1**:779-782

[7] Kaplan DH, Shankaran V, Dighe AS, Stockert E, Aguet M, Old LJ, et al. Demonstration of an interferon gamma-dependent tumor surveillance system in immunocompetent mice. Proceedings of the National Academy of Sciences of the United States of America. 1998;**95**:7556-7561

[8] Shankaran V, Ikeda H, Bruce AT, White JM, Swanson PE, Old LJ, et al. IFNgamma and lymphocytes prevent primary tumour development and shape tumour immunogenicity. Nature. 2001;**410**:1107-1111

[9] Talpaz M, McCredie KB, Mavligit GM, Gutterman JU. Leukocyte interferon-induced myeloid cytoreduction in chronic myelogenous leukemia. Blood. 1983;**62**:689-692

[10] Van der Bruggen P, Traversari C, Chomez P, et al. A gene encoding an antigen recognized by cytolytic T lymphocytes on a human melanoma. Science. 1991;**254**(5038):1643-1647

[11] Karbach J, Neumann A, Atmaca A, et al. Efficient in vivo priming by vaccination with recombinant NY-ESO-1 protein and CpG in antigen naive prostate cancer patients. Clinical Cancer Research. 2011;**17**(4):861-870

[12] Parkhurst MR, Fitzgerald EB, Southwood S, Sette A, Rosenberg SA, Kawakami Y. Identification of a shared HLA-A*0201-restricted T-cell epitope from the melanoma antigen tyrosinase-related protein 2 (TRP2). Cancer Research. 1998;**58**(21):4895-4901

[13] DeFilippis RA, Goodwin EC, Wu L, DiMaio D. Endogenous human papillomavirus E6 and E7 proteins differentially regulate proliferation, senescence, and apoptosis in HeLa cervical carcinoma cells. Journal of Virology. 2003;**77**(2):1551-1563

[14] Kash N, Lee MA, Kollipara R, Downing C, Guidry J, Tyring SK. Safety and efficacy data on vaccines and immunization to human papillomavirus. Journal of Clinical Medicine. 2015;**4**(4):614-633

[15] Roden R, Wu TC. How will HPV vaccines affect cervical cancer? Nature Reviews. Cancer. 2006;**6**:753-763

[16] Chang MH, Chen CJ, Lai MS, Hsu HM, Wu TC, Kong MS, et al. Universal hepatitis B vaccination in Taiwan and the incidence of hepatocellular carcinoma in children. Taiwan childhood Hepatoma study group. The New England Journal of Medicine. 1997;**336**(26):1855-1859

[17] Higano CS, Schellhammmer PF, Small EJ, et al. Integrated data from 2 randomized, double-blind,

placebo-controlled, phase 3 trials of active cellular immunotherapy with sipuleucel-T in advanced prostate cancer. Cancer. 2009;**115**:3670-3679

[18] Kantoff PW, Higano CS, Shore ND, et al. Sipuleucel-T immunotherapy for castration-resistant prostate cancer. The New England Journal of Medicine. 2010;**363**(5):411-422

[19] Obeid J, Hu Y, Slingluff CL Jr. Vaccines, adjuvants, and dendritic cell activators-current status and future challenges. Seminars in Oncology. 2015;**42**(4):549-561

[20] Mach N, Gillessen S, Wilson SB, Sheehan C, Mihm M, Dranoff G. Differences in dendritic cells stimulated in vivo by tumors engineered to secrete granulocyte macrophage colony-stimulating factor or Flt3-ligand. Cancer Research. 2000;**60**(12):3239-3246

[21] Manjili MH, Wang XY, MacDonald IJ, Arnouk H, Yang GY, Pritchard MT, et al. Cancer immunotherapy and heat-shock proteins: Promises and challenges. Expert Opinion on Biological Therapy;**4**(3):363-373

[22] Rosenberg SA, Restifo NP. Adoptive cell transfer as personalized immunotherapy for human cancer. Science. 2015;**348**(6230):62-68

[23] Rohaan MW, Wilgenhof S, Haanen JBAG. Adoptive cellular therapies: The current landscape. Virchows Archiv. 2019;**474**(4):449-461

[24] Verdegaal EM. Adoptive cell therapy: A highly successful individualized therapy for melanoma with great potential for other malignancies. Current Opinion in Immunology. 2016;**39**:90-95

[25] Brudno JN, Somerville RP, Shi V, et al. Allogeneic T cells that express an anti-CD19 chimeric antigen receptor induce remissions of B-cell malignancies that Progress after allogeneic hematopoietic stem-cell transplantation without causing graft-versus-host disease. Journal of Clinical Oncology. 2016;**34**(10):1112-1121

[26] Kochenderfer JN, Dudley ME, Kassim SH, et al. Chemotherapy refractory diffuse large B-cell lymphoma and indolent B-cell malignancies can be effectively treated with autologous T cells expressing an anti-CD19 chimeric antigen receptor. Journal of Clinical Oncology. 2015;**33**(6):540-549

[27] Maude SL, Frey N, Shaw PA, et al. Chimeric antigen receptor T cells for sustained remissions in leukemia. The New England Journal of Medicine. 2014;**371**(16):1507-1517

[28] Pang Y, Hou X, Yang C, Liu Y, Jiang G. Advances on chimeric antigen receptor-modified T-cell therapy for oncotherapy. Molecular Cancer. 2018;**17**(1):91

[29] Ljunggren HG, Karre K. In search of the 'missing self': MHC molecules and NK cell recognition. Immunology Today. 1990;**11**:237-244

[30] Ruggeri L, Capanni M, Casucci M, et al. Role of natural killer cell alloreactivity in HLA-mismatched hematopoietic stem cell transplantation. Blood. 1999;**94**(1):333-339

[31] Coulson A, Levy A, Gossell-Williams M. Monoclonal antibodies in cancer therapy: Mechanisms, successes and limitations. The West Indian Medical Journal. 2014;**63**(6):650-654

[32] Vanneman M, Dranoff G. Combining immunotherapy and targeted therapies in cancer treatment. Nature Reviews. Cancer. 2012;**12**(4):237-251

[33] Pinto AC, Ades F, de Azambuja E, Piccart-Gebhart M. Trastuzumab for patients with HER2 positive breast cancer: Delivery, duration and combination therapies. Breast. 2013;**22**(Suppl 2):S152-S155

[34] Steiner M, Neri D. Antibody-radionuclide conjugates for cancer therapy: Historical considerations and new trends. Clinical Cancer Research. 2011;**17**(20):6406-6416

[35] Flygare JA, Pillow TH, Aristoff P. Antibody-drug conjugates for the treatment of cancer. Chemical Biology and Drug Design. 2013;**81**(1):113-121

[36] Sharma P, Allison JP. Immune checkpoint targeting in cancer therapy: Toward combination strategies with curative potential. Cell. 2015;**161**(2):205-214

[37] Tsai HF, Hsu PN. Cancer immunotherapy by targeting immune checkpoints: Mechanism of T cell dysfunction in cancer immunity and new therapeutic targets. Journal of Biomedical Science. 2017;**24**(1):35

[38] Postow MA, Chesney J, Pavlick AC, et al. Nivolumab and ipilimumab versus ipilimumab in untreated melanoma. The New England Journal of Medicine. 2015;**372**(21):2006-2017

[39] Langer CJ, Gadgeel SM, Borghaei H, et al. Carboplatin and pemetrexed with or without pembrolizumab for advanced, non-squamous nonsmall-cell lung cancer: A randomised, phase 2 cohort of the open-label KEYNOTE-021 study. The Lancet Oncology. 2016;**17**(11):1497-1508

[40] Hodi FS, O'Day SJ, McDermott DF, et al. Improved survival with ipilimumab in patients with metastatic melanoma. The New England Journal of Medicine. 2010;**363**(8):711-723

[41] Corsello SM, Barnabei A, Marchetti P, Vecchis LD, Salvatori R, Torino F. Endocrine side effects induced by immune checkpoint inhibitors. The Journal of Clinical Endocrinology and Metabolism. 2013;**98**(4):1361-1375

[42] Di Giacomo AM, Biagioli M, Maio M. The emerging toxicity profiles of anti-CTLA-4 antibodies across clinical indications. Seminars in Oncology. 2010;**37**:499-507

Chapter 2

Cancer Vaccines

Carmen Murias Henriquez, Hendrik-Tobias Arkenau, Valérie Dutoit and Anna Patrikidou

Abstract

Recent advances in immuno-oncology have allowed for the design of more specific and efficient cancer vaccine approaches. There has been an improvement in molecular biology techniques, as well as a greater understanding of the mechanisms involved in the activation and regulation of T cells and the interplay between the components of the immune system and the escape mechanisms used by cancer cells and the tumour microenvironment. As a result, many interesting developments in therapeutic cancer vaccines are ongoing, with influence on survival still to be proven. The spectrum of tumour antigens that are recognised by T cells is still largely unchartered and, most importantly, dynamically evolving over time, driven by clonal evolution and treatment-driven selection. Vaccine approaches currently in development and tested in clinical studies are based on tumour antigens specifically identified for each tumour type, on tumour cells or dendritic cells, the latter having the potential to be modified to incorporate immunostimulatory genes. However, interplay between the immune system and the tumour and the inhibitory mechanisms developed by tumour cells to subvert immune responses are crucial issues that will need to be targeted in order for efficient therapeutic vaccines to emerge.

Keywords: vaccine, T cells, tumour antigens, immune system

1. Introduction

Cancer constitutes one of the biggest burdens in the Western society with lung, breast, prostate and colorectal cancer being the most prevalent. Despite declining rates in the Western societies [1], there have been an estimated 9.6 million deaths by cancer worldwide in 2018 [2, 3], and it is expected that this number will further increase over time.

The molecular nature of human cancers is complex and varies among tumours and individuals. For that reason, the approach towards a more personalised cancer treatment has gained intense interest. Treatment approaches are being increasingly changing from histology- to molecular-based therapies, including targeting the interplay between cancer and the immune system.

In the last few decades, major advances have been made in recognising that an effective immune system—or the lack thereof—plays an important role in cancer development, growth and metastasis. For example, the presence of tumour-infiltrating lymphocytes (TILs) has been identified as a positive prognostic factor in multiple cancer types [4]. Utilising the body's defences and reactivating the antitumour immune response, initially regarded as a simple paradigm, have created a scientific and therapeutic revolution [5]. After decades of attempts, immunotherapy has achieved a major breakthrough with the sensational successes of immunomodulation with checkpoint blockade (i.e. PD-1/PD-L1 and CTLA-4 inhibitors, among others). In addition to that, the recent development of immune effector cell therapy in the form of chimeric antigen receptor T cells for haematological malignancies has opened exciting horizons for solid tumours as well [6, 7]. Up to now, therapeutic vaccination against cancer, despite few examples like Bacillus Calmette-Guérin (BCG) treatment for superficial bladder cancer [8], the oncolytic virus-based talimogene laherparepvec (T-VEC) [9] and the Sipuleucel vaccine in prostate cancer [10], has not achieved similar results.

Nevertheless, new vaccine development techniques as well as immunotherapy combination strategies shape the pipeline of current trial development and represent a promise and challenge for the future.

1.1 The T-cell response to cancer

The immune system and in particular dendritic cells (DCs) and macrophages are capable, to a variable extent, to recognise damage-associated molecular patterns (DAMPs), thus eliciting an innate immune response. The major DAMP driving innate host antitumour immune responses is tumour-derived DNA, which is detected via the stimulator of interferon gene (STING) pathway and results in type I IFN production [11].

The adaptive immune response begins when cancer antigens are presented to T and B cells by DCs. Although B-cell responses are probably playing a role in antitumour immunity, not much is yet known about them [12]. The following text will therefore mostly refer to antitumour T-cell responses. Tumour antigens are transported via lymphatic vessels to the lymph nodes, where they are captured by lymph node-resident DCs. Alternatively, tissue-resident DCs capture antigens at the tumour site and migrate to induce T-cell responses in the lymph node [13]. DCs present protein antigens in the context of major histocompatibility complex (MHC) class I and II molecules, allowing the stimulation of rare antigen-specific $CD8^+$ or $CD4^+$ T lymphocytes, respectively. Upon antigen encounter, CD8 T cells differentiate into cytotoxic T lymphocytes (CTLs) that have tumour-killing capacities, whereas CD4 T cells will provide CD8 T-cell help [13]. CD4 T cells can also be induced to become $FoxP3^+$ regulatory T cells (Tregs), which are then able to inhibit antitumoural immune responses [14].

A tumour mass is not composed solely of tumour cells, but contains immune cells, stromal cells and vessels, a concept known as the tumour microenvironment. Tumours are organised in various reciprocal, local and systemic relations with myeloid and lymphoid immune cell populations, both being key factors in regulating immune responses to cancer. During progression, tumours are able to modulate the immune response and highjack it to their advantage, in order to invade and grow. Macrophages can be polarised to a pro-tumoural and anti-inflammatory (called M2) phenotype at the tumour's advantage. In addition, myeloid-derived suppressor cells (MDCSs) accumulate in the tumour microenvironment and are able to suppress antitumour T-cell responses [15, 16].

1.2 The three phases of tumour immunoediting: elimination, equilibrium and escape

The principles of cancer immunoediting have set the basis for understanding the dual host-protective and immuno-sculpting effects of immunity on cancer [17]. During cancer immunoediting, the host immune system influences tumour fate in three phases through activation of innate and adaptive immune mechanisms: elimination, equilibrium and escape.

1.2.1 Elimination

The elimination phase occurs when cancer cells are eradicated by a competent immune system. This is evidenced by immunodeficient mice that have an increased propensity to develop carcinogen-induced and spontaneous cancers than wild-type mice [18]. In addition, tumours that come from immunodeficient mice are more immunogenic than those from immunocompetent mice, as they have not been edited by the immune response. Patients suffering from AIDS [19] or being under immunosuppression are similarly more prone to develop cancer [20, 21]. The role of CD8 T cells has been more extensively studied; however interplay with CD4 T-cell responses is also required in order to have an integrated and efficient response [22, 23].

1.2.2 Equilibrium

The sporadic tumour cells that survive immune destruction will enter into the equilibrium phase where editing arises. Immune pressure is mostly mediated by CD4 and CD8 T cells [24]. Upon tumour editing, more mutations will be acquired, which will favour entry into the escape phase of immunoediting. Importantly, the process of incomplete elimination promotes the generation of tumour cell variants with decreased immunogenicity [23]. The identification of hidden cancer cells in an equilibrium state remains a challenge; however, advances in technology and biomarkers may allow for circulating tumour cells and niches to be investigated further.

1.2.3 Escape

The escape phase represents the final phase of the process, where immunologically sculpted tumours begin to grow progressively, becoming clinically apparent. Tumour escape can result from many different mechanisms including reduced immune recognition, through loss of MHC class I, co-stimulatory molecules or tumour antigens. In addition, the tumour induces many molecules and cells to induce an immunosuppressive tumour microenvironment. Cytokines such as VEGF and TGF-β, immunoregulatory molecules such as indoleamine 2,3-dioxygenase (IDO), programmed death-ligand 1 (PD-L1) and ligands for Tim3 and lymphocyte-activation gene 3 (LAG-3), among others, are induced to supress the incoming CD4 and CD8 T cells. In addition, many cellular components of the tumour microenvironment, such as macrophages and neutrophils, are being redirected in an anti-inflammatory pro-tumoural state [25–27].

1.3 The principles and means of immunotherapy

Although cancer cells have the unique ability to escape from the immune response, the knowledge that immune cells are able to recognise tumours allows development of therapies that utilise the immune system [28]. Cancer immunotherapies focus on exploiting both the innate and adaptive arms of the immune system. They can be classified into vaccines, monoclonal antibodies (including immune checkpoint inhibitors), recombinant cytokines, small molecules and adoptive T-cell transfer, including chimeric antigen receptor (CAR), TCR and TIL therapy [29–32].

1.3.1 Vaccines

The aim of cancer vaccination is to prime cellular immune response against tumour-specific antigens. Despite its limitations mainly owing to heterogeneous tumour antigen composition and expression and their susceptibility to various mechanisms of immune suppression, it is being intensively developed. Currently revisited with strategies aiming at combinations with other immunotherapies, cancer vaccines will be addressed in detail in this chapter.

1.3.2 Monoclonal antibodies

Antibodies target (a) factors that regulate signal pathways used by cancer cells in division and angiogenesis (such as the VEGF inhibitor bevacizumab) [33]; (b) tumour-associated antigens, activating antibody-dependent cellular cytotoxicity (such as the Her2-directed antibody trastuzumab) [34]; (c) complement-dependent cytotoxicity (such as the anti-20 and anti-EGFR antibodies rituximab and cetuximab); and (d) immune blockade with checkpoint inhibitors such as anti-CTLA4 antibodies (ipilimumab and tremelimumab), anti-PD1 antibodies (nivolumab and pembrolizumab) or anti-PD-L1 antibodies (atezolizumab, durvalumab, and avelumab) [31].

1.3.3 Recombinant cytokines

Immunostimulatory recombinant cytokines promote lymphocyte activation via control of transcriptional and metabolic programmes [35]. An example is recombinant IL-2 (aldesleukin, Proleukin®) that has been used to treat renal cancer and melanoma [36]. Another recombinant cytokine approved by the US Food and Drug Administration (FDA) for the adjuvant treatment in resected melanoma patients is pegylated interferon α-2β (Sylatron®), a member of the IFN cytokine family [37]. Concurrent administration of immunostimulatory cytokines such as IL-2 and granulocyte-macrophage colony-stimulating factor (GM-CSF) may also enhance the efficacy of antibody therapy [38]. Limitations include their antigenicity, poor pharmacokinetics and high toxicity [29].

1.3.4 Small molecules

The use of small molecules in cancer immunotherapy has been increasing, given their ability to target both intracellular and surface targets. Plerixafor is a small molecule that inhibits the binding interaction of stromal cell-derived factor 1 (SDF-1) to the chemokine receptor CXCR4, used as a haematopoietic stem cell mobiliser [39]. This small molecule aims to prevent the development of cancer metastasis in cancer patients, principally in pancreatic ductal adenocarcinoma patients [29]. Another known small molecule called imiquimod, used for the treatment of basal cell carcinoma, is an agonist for toll-like receptor (TLR)-7. Imiquimod-mediated TLR7 activation induces production of proinflammatory cytokines, inhibits Tregs and induces activation of natural killer (NK) cells to eliminate cancer cells [29]. IDO inhibitors are being tested as well in multiple malignancies, but results as monotherapy have been disappointing [40]. Combinations with other immunotherapeutic agents or with chemotherapy/radiation are being currently investigated. A much anticipated combination, however, of the small molecule IDO1 inhibitor with pembrolizumab failed to provide significant benefit in a phase 3 trial in unresectable or metastatic melanoma [41]. Finally, ongoing research evaluates the adenosine signalling with adenosine receptor inhibitors [42].

1.3.5 Adoptive T-cell therapy

The use of cancer patient's own immune effector cells is a novel cancer immunotherapy, also called adoptive cell therapy. Starting with TILs, it has moved to the generation of artificial T cells that are genetically altered to express an antitumour antibody (CARs) or a selected TCR [30]. These cells are multiplied and subsequently transferred back to the patient, who usually receives conditioning chemotherapy. TIL therapy has shown some clinical evidence of efficacy in the treatment of melanoma [43] and cervical cancer [44], with the LN-145 TIL therapy recently obtaining breakthrough therapy designation by FDA, while its potential is being further investigated. Generation of tumour-specific T cells through expression of a TCR that has shown antitumour properties is ongoing for several malignancies [44]. CAR T cells, which are engineered to express part of a tumour-specific antibody, linked to intracellular T-cell signalling domains are gaining major interest [45]. Two anti-CD19 CAR T-cell therapies have so far received FDA approval in haematological malignancies, notably tisagenlecleucel for diffuse large B-cell lymphoma (DLBCL) and acute lymphoblastic leukaemia and axicabtagene ciloleucel for primary or transformed DLBCL, mediastinal and high-grade B-cell lymphoma [46]. Research on CAR T-cell therapies in solid malignancies is currently ongoing.

2. Cancer vaccines

2.1 Introduction

Cancer vaccination seeks to generate, amplify or skew (or the combination thereof) antitumour immunity. In order to reach such an ambitious goal, many approaches are in development, including the administration of tumour antigens, often with antigen presenting cells or other immune modulators.

Current technological advances in genomics, data science and cancer immunotherapy enable the fast mapping of alterations within a genome, as well as the rational selection of vaccine targets and on-demand production of a therapy that has been customised to a patient's individual tumour. With the development of vaccination being promoted by emerging innovations in the digital era, vaccinating patients according to their individual tumour mutational profile may become the first truly personalised treatment for cancer.

It is important to distinguish vaccines that are designed to prevent cancer from the ones that are designed to treat cancer. The mode of action of the HPV vaccine for the prevention of cervical and other HPV-associated cancers [9] and of hepatitis B virus (HBV) vaccine for the prevention of HBV infection that carries a risk of development of hepatocellular carcinoma [47] is the prevention of infection itself. Their action is based on the generation of antiviral antibodies and has led to a net reduction in the incidence of these cancers in vaccinated individuals [48]. The development of therapeutic cancer vaccines has been more challenging. The nature of the antigen, which, in the case of therapeutic cancer vaccines, is derived from self-antigens against which the host has been tolerised and the presence of a hostile tumour microenvironment are key limiting factors.

2.2 Therapeutic vaccines

2.2.1 FDA-approved vaccines

Three therapeutic cancer vaccines have been approved by the FDA. The Bacillus Calmette-Guérin (BCG, TheraCys®, TICE®) vaccine, based on a live attenuated strain of *Mycobacterium bovis*, was the first approved cancer vaccine for use in non-muscle invasive bladder carcinoma following transurethral resection. It showed a prolongation in disease-free survival (DFS) of 30 months in patients with bladder carcinoma in situ (CIS) and of 22.5 months in patients with Ta/T1 urothelial carcinoma compared to 4.9 months in bladder CIS and 10.5 months in Ta/T1 patients treated with topical doxorubicin [49].

Sipuleucel-T (Provenge) is an autologous DC vaccine for patients with minimally symptomatic or asymptomatic metastatic castrate-resistant prostate cancer (mCRPC). Patient's DCs are being injected with a recombinant fusion protein, PA2024, which consists of a tumour antigen, the prostate acid phosphatase (PAP) and GM-CSF, before reinfusion. The phase 3 IMPACT study, a double-blind, placebo-controlled, phase 3 trial of 512 mCRPC patients randomised to receive either three infusions of Sipuleucel-T or placebo 2 weeks apart, demonstrated statistically significant improvement of 4.1 months in median overall survival (OS) (25.8 months in the Sipuleucel-T group compared to 21.7 months in the placebo group) [10]. However, this study elicited significant criticism in regard with the observed—albeit modest—OS benefit without correlation with a progression-free survival (PFS) benefit or a T-cell response, the lack of association between survival benefit and T-cell proliferation responses, the fact that T-cell proliferative responses to the chimeric antigen (PA2024) did not cross-react to the physiological human PAP and hence the absence of alternative mechanisms to explain the survival benefit [50].

The third approved vaccine, called talimogene laherparepvec (T-VEC or Imlygic), is an oncolytic herpes virus 1-based vaccine for advanced melanoma. In this vaccine, two viral genes governing neurovirulence and blockade of antigen presentation are deleted, and the virus is modified to produce GM-CSF to enhance immunogenicity [8]. T-VEC was approved based on data published on the phase 3 OPTiM trial. The vaccine virus, injected intralesionally, infects both the cancer and normal cells but can only replicate within cancer cells. The OPTiM trial showed more durable response rate ($\geq$6 months) with T-VEC than GM-CSF alone, as well as higher overall response rate and a longer median OS (23.3 months compared to 18.9 months with GM-CSF alone) in patients with stage IIIB, IIIC or IV M1a melanoma [51].

2.2.2 Mode of action of therapeutic vaccines

The mode of action of most therapeutic vaccines involves development of cell-mediated immunity directed against tumour antigens; such antigens ought to ideally not be expressed in normal cells or have restricted normal expression, be of high expression on cancer cells, be highly immunogenic and be necessary for cancer cell survival [32]. Tumour antigens can be delivered as peptides, proteins, DNA or viral vectors or tumour cells themselves. They are usually administered with an adjuvant (see Section 2.5), in order to potentiate the immune response. Tumour antigens can also be generated via antigen spreading, which is the exposure of novel antigens after an initial antitumour response [52].

2.3 Tumour antigens

2.3.1 Tumour-associated antigens (TAAs)

TAAs are self-antigens commonly expressed in a specific tumour type among different patients. They are derived from non-mutated proteins that are overexpressed in tumour cells as compared to normal cells. The first TAAs were discovered after the cloning of gene-encoding proteins that generated epitopes recognised by tumour reactive TILs [53]. The first gene discovered that was reported to encode a tumour antigen recognised by T cells was MAGE-1 [53]. Since the discovery of MAGE-1, a large number of TAAs have been described, and they are classified into shared TAAs and unique TAAs [54], the latter being present only in individual patients.

Shared TAAs can be classified in three main groups, cancer/testis antigens, overexpressed antigens and differentiation antigens [54].

Cancer testis antigens (*CT*) are a large family of TAAs expressed in human tumours of different histological origins but not in normal adult tissues, with the exception of immune-privileged cells such as testis and placenta [55]. These antigens result from the reactivation of genes that are normally silent in adult tissues but that are transcriptionally activated in tumours. This quasi-exclusive tumour-restricted expression pattern (sparing normal germ cells that do not express HLA class I molecules) as well as their high prevalence make them ideal vaccine candidates [55]. They have been identified and tested in many human clinical trials [56]; however, there is usually very little knowledge about their specific function, especially with regard to tumour transformation. CT antigens include, among others, the MAGE-A, MAGE-B, MAGE-C, NY-ESO and SSX-2 families.

Overexpressed antigens are expressed at a higher level in tumour cells than in normal tissues. Expression of these antigens at variable levels in normal cells conveys the risk of autoimmune attack upon vaccination, but a large number of clinical trials have used these antigens with up to now few side effects [57]. Some examples of this group of antigens are tumour suppressor proteins such as p53 and the antiapoptotic proteins hTERT and Mucin 1 (MUC-1).

Tissue-specific (cell lineage) differentiation antigens are shared between the tumour and the normal tissue of origin, albeit with variable specificity. They include carcinoembryonic antigen (CEA), prostate-specific antigen (PSA), HER2/neu and melanoma lineage antigens such as gp-100, Melan-A/Mart-1 and tyrosinase, expressed in melanoma [58]. As for overexpressed antigens, they are endowed with a risk for autoimmune reactions.

The advantage of TAAs is that they are frequently expressed by the majority of patients and can therefore be used to treat many patients. The disadvantage of TAAs is the fact that some of them retain a level of expression in normal tissues, entailing the potential risk of autoimmune damage upon efficient vaccination. In addition, as TAAs derive from self-antigens, specific T cells have undergone negative selection, leaving only T cells with low avidity of antigen recognition, which are not able to generate strong immune responses.

2.3.2 Tumour-specific antigens (TSAs)

TSAs are antigens resulting from point mutations. They represent neoantigens mostly expressed by individual tumours. TSAs are tumour-specific, and it is usually viewed that their immunogenicity is not restricted by central tolerance, which is true when the mutated epitope is different enough from the wild-type one. Additionally, induced T-cell responses are not expected to result in autoimmune toxicity [59]. Moreover, neoantigens may be more resistant to immune selection, as they are critical for the oncogenic process and, therefore, essential for keeping the neoplastic state. In contrast, the fact that TSAs are patient-specific prevents broad vaccination and requires identification in a patient-specific manner. However, recent availability of sequencing technologies and epitope prediction algorithms allows for a rapid identification of potential neoantigens. Methods of in silico prediction of neo-epitope candidates with a high potential for neoantigen generation potentially present in multiple patients. These neoantigens hold the potential for development of "off the shelf" T-cell therapies, aiming to complement individualised, patient- and tumour-specific precision medicine approaches [32]. Nevertheless, it should be kept in mind that only a small percentage of mutations are being presented on MHC molecules at the tumour cell surface, making verification of the presence of a neo-epitope at the tumour cell surface a prerequisite [60, 61].

2.4 Types of vaccines

2.4.1 Peptide vaccines

Peptide vaccines consist in the delivery of MHC class I- or class II-restricted peptide epitopes derived from tumour antigens with the intent of activating $CD8^+$ and $CD4^+$ T cells. As peptides are not immunogenic per se, they need to be injected with an adjuvant [62]. GM-CSF, Montanide and TLR agonists, among others, have shown clinical benefit in small- and larger-scale clinical trials [63–65]. Peptide vaccines have the limitation of being applicable only to patients that have the HLA allele the peptide is restricted to. In addition, most vaccines are made of MHC class I-restricted peptides, therefore not eliciting CD4 T-cell help [66, 67]. In order to overcome this issue, the addition of non-tumour-specific peptides has been used, but limited data is available on the improvement provided by such heterologous helper peptides [68]. Overall, the numerous clinical trials performed in different tumour types have not provided satisfactory results yet [69].

Using multiple peptides derived from different TAAs targeting several antigens at once could overcome such tumour escape mechanisms. This multipeptide approach has demonstrated in in vitro and in vivo studies that multiple peptides do not compete for MHC presentation, inducing a multi-specific T-cell response [70–72]. The use of synthetic peptides with improved DC-targeting mechanisms, such as integrating pattern recognition receptors or TLRs [73], the conjugation of synthetic peptides to a DC-targeting antibody [74] or the encapsulation of long peptides in structures such as nanoparticles, liposomes or nano-hydrogel systems to enhance T-cell priming by DCs [75, 76] are some of the strategies under investigation towards a more efficient processing and presentation pathway that would lead to greater T-cell activation.

In two trials (a phase 1 and a randomised phase 2) combining single-dose pre-vaccine cyclophosphamide with IMA901, a renal cell carcinoma (RCC) peptide vaccine containing 10 antigens (9 HLA class I-binding and 1 HLA class II-binding) adjuvanted with GM-CSF in HLA-$A02^+$ subjects showed that there was an improvement in survival with amplification of antigenic response and a reduction in suppressive circulatory T cells and MDSCs, with a disease control rate (DCR) at 6 months of 31% (95% CI: 3–35%) [77]. Mouse models also support combinations of multipeptide vaccines and chemotherapy. However, the addition of IMA901 to first-line sunitinib (an anti-angiogenic tyrosine kinase inhibitor) failed to show improvement in metastatic renal cancer, owing to low-level immune responses [78], despite the fact that sunitinib has been shown to decrease the number of Tregs in mice and patients with RCC [79, 80], as well as MDSCs in patients with RCC [81].

Owing to their tumour specificity, much effort has been made in order to exploit neoantigens for vaccine development. Such neoantigen-directed vaccines have been developed for melanoma, using either synthetic RNAs containing up to 10 predicted neoantigens or long peptides targeting up to 20 neoantigens [82, 83]. In these trials, neo-epitopes were chosen to bind HLA class I [82] or HLA class I and II molecules [83] and showed activation of $CD4^+$ and $CD8^+$ T cells in response to vaccination.

Peptide vaccines can also be helpful in the prevention of the progression of a premalignant lesion to cancer. The MUC-1 peptide vaccine has been tested as a prevention of progression of colon adenoma to colorectal cancer [84]. MUC-1 was highly immunogenic in about half of the patients evaluated. Moreover, response to the vaccine correlated with prevaccination levels of circulating MDSCs, as nonresponders had a significantly higher percentage of MDSCs ($p < 0.05$); interestingly, no such association was observed for regulatory T cells.

NeuVax is a peptide vaccine that has been developed for early-stage node-positive low or intermediate HER2-expressing breast cancer after standard of care treatment [85]. The vaccine is composed of a peptide isolated from HER2/neu proto-oncogene combined with GM-CSF. Final results of a phase 1/2 clinical trial showed a non-significant improvement in 5-year DFS of 89.7% in the vaccine group versus 80.2% in the control group ($p = 0.08$); the improvement in DFS was even greater in the sub-group of optimally dosed patients (94.6%; $p = 0.05$ versus the control group) [86]. The vaccine is now being tested in an ongoing phase 3 trial (NCT01479244).

CDX-110 is a peptide vaccine also known as the rindopepimut vaccine. It is a 14-mer peptide covering the EGFRvIII mutation (the commonest form of EGFR mutation in human glioblastoma multiforme (GBM), detected in 23–33% of tumours) [87], and it is linked to the adjuvant keyhole limpet hemocyanin (KLH) to stimulate a specific immune response against EGFRvIII expressing tumour cells. This vaccine has been evaluated in three phase 2 clinical trials (ACTIVATE, ACT II and ACT III trials) for newly diagnosed GBM and one phase 2 (ReACT trial) for recurrent GBM. The ACTIVATE trial demonstrated that patients with EGFRvIII-specific humoral responses had an improved median OS as compared to patients not displaying immune responses (47.7 months vs. 22.8 months OS) [88]. The ACT II and ACT III clinical trials demonstrated longer PFS and OS than with historically matched controls [88, 89]. Deceivingly, the phase 3 trial ACT IV for newly diagnosed GBM was terminated for futility at the second preplanned interim analysis (HR: 0.99 for rindopepimut versus control, 95% CI: 0.74–1.31) [90]. A lack of benefit was also observed in the intention-to-treat population. The study confirmed earlier-phase trial findings of rindopepimut-induced EGFRvIII-specific antibody responses in the majority of patients; however, the fact that loss of EGFRvIII was observed in patients receiving or not the vaccine suggests that this target is unstable and therefore not a suitable antigen for immunotherapy. The phase 2 ReACT trial, evaluating the combination of bevacizumab and rindopepimut for recurrent GBM, showed that the vaccine induced robust anti-EGFRvIII antibodies in the majority of patients. The primary endpoint of PFS at 6 months was improved for the rindopepimut arm, albeit non-significantly (28% vs. 16%, $p = 0.12$), with a similar outcome for OS and duration of response. Rapid anti-EGFRvIII antibody generation was shown to be associated with prolonged OS in the rindopepimut arm [91]. A major criticism for this study, which could explain the non-significant results, is that the EGFRvIII status was principally decided on diagnostic tumour specimens, despite the known fact that EGFRvIII expression is lost in half of tumours upon recurrence.

2.4.2 DC vaccines

In order to improve peptide presentation in vivo, cancer vaccines using DC have been developed. DC-based vaccines are safe and immunogenic, and they have the ability to promote clinically significant tumour regression in some patients [92–94]. Clinical trials performed with DC-based vaccines usually involve an individualised patient vaccination approach with single clinical trial arms, which makes it difficult to evoke firm conclusions about their efficacy. Several cells such as monocytes and $CD34^+$ progenitor cells, antigens including complex tumour lysates and synthetic MHC class I-restricted peptides have all been used in different trials [95]. Some promising and important clinical trials involving DC vaccines have been published. Sipuleucel-T (Provenge) is one of the three FDA-approved vaccines (see Section 2.2.1). In addition to the IMPACT trial that led to FDA approval, 42 men with localised prostate cancer received Sipuleucel-T in a phase 2 study prior to radical prostatectomy [96]. Increased incidence of T cells was observed in the post-operative prostate gland histology compared to preoperative biopsies. Currently, clinical trials are investigating combination of Sipuleucel-T with other approved drugs, such as abiraterone acetate, enzalutamide, radium-223, ipilimumab and atezolizumab (NCT01487863, NCT01981122, NCT02463799, NCT01832870, NCT01804465, and NCT3024216).

A clinical trial that used DCs loaded with a MUC-1-derived peptide and heterologous pan DR epitope (PADRE) peptides (universal CD4 T-cell helper peptides) delivered subcutaneously in patients with RCC has shown encouraging objective clinical responses and immunologic responses [97]. A phase 1/2 clinical trial used autologous WT-1 (Wilms' tumour 1, a shared TAA) mRNA-loaded DCs in patients with acute myeloid leukaemia (AML) in remission after standard of care, with the aim of eradicating or controlling residual disease. This study showed clinical responses correlating with increased WT-1-specific $CD8^+$ T-cell frequencies, as well as elevated levels of post-vaccine-activated NK cells [98]. Another study used patient-derived AML cells fused with autologous DCs vaccination in post-chemotherapy remission AML patients, achieving a marked rise in circulating T cells recognising whole AML cells and leukaemia-specific antigens that persisted for more than 6 months, which was associated with prolonged survival [99].

DCVax is a DC vaccine that has been developed for GBM. Two phase 1/2 studies tested the vaccine, which collectively recruited 39 patients, 20 of whom had newly diagnosed GBM and the remaining had recurrent high-grade glioma [100, 101]. For the newly diagnosed patients, the median OS with the addition of DC vaccine to the standard of care chemoradiation was 36 months. Long-term survival was also reported for some patients; 33% of patients reached or exceeded a 4-year survival, 27% reached an OS of 6 years, and two patients achieved a 10-year survival. The first report of the DCVax 2:1 randomised phase 3 trial in newly diagnosed GBM unfortunately does not allow interpretation as it is endowed with methodological flaws [102].

Some findings have suggested that the current DC vaccines can be optimised in order to get improved clinical outcomes. The discovery that the overexpression of CD40L in human DCs produces an increased stimulation of the T-cell response to tumour antigens such as gp100 and Melan-A is promising [103]. Additionally, DC function can be enhanced by stimulating antigen-specific Th1 and CTL responses through modulation of other co-stimulatory or co-inhibitory molecules, such as PD-1, CTLA4, CD28, OX40, etc. [104, 105]. On the contrary, suppressing the ubiquitin-editing enzyme A20 or the scavenger receptor SRA/CD204 in human DC helps in the development of IFN-α-producing Th1 cells and antigen-specific $CD8^+$ T cells [106, 107]. These developments suggest that there is promising data for the future in DC-based cancer vaccines.

2.4.3 Tumour cell vaccines

Tumours concentrate a high number of genetic modifications in somatic cells and therefore carry a large number of potential antigens. For that reason, vaccination with whole tumour cells has been an interesting strategy, with the limitation that they need to be patient-tailored. Autologous tumour cell vaccines have been evaluated in several cancer types such as lung cancer [108], melanoma [109, 110], RCC [111], prostate cancer [112] and colorectal cancer [113, 114]. In order to prepare the vaccine, a large amount of tumour tissue needs to be collected, which impedes its application in some tumour types or some individuals.

MVX-ONCO-1 is an autologous tumour cell vaccine containing irradiated tumour cells from a patient and a capsule implanted with a genetically modified allogeneic cell line that continuously releases the adjuvant GM-CSF [115]. Results of the first-in-human phase 1 trial testing of this vaccine reported an excellent safety profile, the main toxicity being a discomfort at the implantation site (20%) [116].

Over 50% of patients (8/15) experienced either partial response (PR) or stable disease (SD) including disappearance of lung metastases, with interesting activity in head and neck squamous cell carcinoma (HNSCC) and chordoma [117]. A phase 2 trial is ongoing in HNSCC (NCT02999646).

Canvaxin was the first allogeneic whole-cell vaccine to be developed and consisted of three melanoma cell lines in combination with BCG as adjuvant [118]. It showed promising results in a phase 2 clinical trial [119, 120], but failed in the randomised phase 3 trial [121]. Although the reasons for the lack of efficiency remain to be determined, it is possible that the induced immune response was not able to control the disease. To potentiate induction of immune response, tumour antigens utilised in vaccines should be linked with potent immunological adjuvants [122]. Such examples are tumour vaccines that have been modified genetically to express co-stimulatory molecules and/or cytokines. Such an example is the GVAX vaccine, an allogeneic whole-cell vaccine modified with the GM-CSF gene, which has been evaluated for recurrent prostate cancer [123, 124], breast cancer [125] and pancreatic cancer [126, 127], but impact on patient survival remains to be proven.

In order to improve the immunogenicity of allogeneic tumour cells, cell lines have been engineered to secrete antisense oligonucleotides to inhibit expression of immunosuppressive cytokines, such as TGF-β. The tumour vaccine Lucanix (Belagenpumatucel-L) has been designed using this strategy to target metastatic NSCLC and has shown significant improvement in OS in two phase 2 clinical trials [128, 129]. However, the phase 3 clinical trial in stage III/IV patients did not demonstrate prolongation of OS in the whole cohort of patients, a survival benefit being however observed in several subgroups of patients [130].

BiovaxID is a patient-specific therapeutic cancer vaccine composed of the patient clonal immunoglobulin molecule idiotype vaccine conjugated to the adjuvant KLH. In a phase 2 clinical trial, the administration of BiovaxID together with GM-CSF in patients diagnosed with follicular lymphoma in complete remission with minimal residual disease demonstrated induction of tumour-specific cellular and humoral immune responses, which translated into clinical benefit, with a median DFS of 8 years and an OS rate of 95% at 9 years [131]. A randomised, controlled phase 3 trial in patients achieving remission after chemotherapy showed a median DFS after randomisation of 44.2 months for the vaccine arm versus 30.6 months for control arm [132]. However, other phase 3 trials failed to demonstrate increase in survival for patients receiving the vaccine [133, 134].

The HyperAcute vaccines are made of tumour cell lines that have been genetically engineered to express the α(1,3)-galactosyltransferase enzyme in order to induce an hyperacute reaction with complement- and antibody-dependant cytotoxicity [135]. They have been tested in several malignancies including melanoma, pancreatic and prostate cancer [136–138] and showed encouraging results improving OS. This vaccine was further evaluated in two phase 3 clinical trials. The IMPRESS study evaluated the vaccine with or without gemcitabine/chemoradiation in resected pancreatic cancer patients but failed to achieve its primary endpoint, with no observed statistically significant difference between the treatment and control groups. The PILLAR trial for borderline resectable (stage II) and advanced unresectable (stage III) pancreatic adenocarcinoma patients, combining the vaccine with FOLFIRINOX or gemcitabine/nab-paclitaxel and chemoradiation, is currently ongoing.

2.4.4 Heat shock protein vaccines

Heat shock proteins (HSPs) are a group of intracellular protein chaperones. Their function is to protect cells from protein misfolding, dysfunction and cell apoptosis, and they have been implicated in the activation of innate and adaptive immunity [139]. Therapeutic HSPs vaccines utilise HSPs as a source of tumour-associated antigens and involve isolation and purification of HSPs from a patient's tumour with subsequent reinfusion of the complex. The advantages of this type of vaccines are, similarly to tumour vaccines, that they do not require a pre-identification of tumour antigens and provide several targets at the same time.

GBM are natural inducers of HSP expression, making them an interesting target for HSP vaccines [139]. A phase 2 trial testing the HSPPC-96 vaccine in recurrent GMB patients showed a 90.2% 6-month OS and a 29.3% 12-month OS, with an interesting observation of an adverse effect of lymphopenia on the vaccination outcome [140]. Adjuvant vaccination following standard treatment by surgery and chemoradiation in patients with newly diagnosed GBM showed a median OS of 23.8 months [141]. Interestingly, this phase 2 trial showed better outcome (median OS: 44.7 months) in patients with low PD-L1-expressing myeloid cells than patients with high PD-L1 myeloid expression (median OS: 18 months) [141]. Nevertheless, a phase II randomised study (Alliance A071101) evaluating the combination of HSPPC-96 vaccine with bevacizumab versus bevacizumab alone in patients with recurrent GBM failed to demonstrate a survival benefit [142]. HSP-based vaccine has also been tested in various malignancies [143].

2.4.5 Viral vectors

Delivery of tumour antigens can be achieved using viral vectors. The advantage of virus-based vaccines is that human immune system has evolved to react efficiently against them with innate and adaptive responses, inducing long-lasting immunity. The most common viruses from which viral vaccines vectors have been developed are poxviruses, adenoviruses and alphaviruses [144]. A potentially restraining factor using viral vectors is the fact that the induced antiviral immune response will neutralise the vector, limiting efficacy of repeated vaccination with the same vector. In order to overcome this, heterologous prime-boost vaccination is used, where initial delivery of a tumour antigen with one virus vector is followed by a boost with the same tumour antigen delivered with another virus vector [145]. Using viral vector also offers the possibility to insert genes coding for adjuvants such as GM-CSF and IL-2.

As an example, the TRICOM vaccine platform exploits heterologous prime-boost vaccination where priming is achieved using a vaccinia vector encoding a chosen TAA and boosting using a fowlpox-derived vector encoding the same TAA. In addition, it incorporates three co-stimulatory molecules for immune activation and has been used in several trials in various malignancies. In men with CRPC, the PROSTVAC vaccine phase 3 trial, using PSA as antigen, failed to positively influence OS [146], although phase 2 trials were encouraging [147, 148]. An analysis of immune response to the PROSTVAC vaccine on pooled data from several clinical trials conducted similarly reported that 68% of the tested patients exhibited evidence of cross-priming with immune responses mounted against TAAs not found in the vaccine, for example, MUC-1, PSMA, PAP and PSCA, a phenomenon known as antigen spreading [149]. Other applications of the TRICOM vaccine in breast and ovarian cancer [150], solid carcinomas [151, 152], colorectal carcinoma [153] or advanced cancers [154] have been tested in phase 1 trials using various antigens and virus vectors, and further studies are planned.

Another example is BN-CV301, a poxvirus-based vaccine that codes for the MUC-1 and CEA TAAs. The phase 1 clinical trial showed no dose-limiting toxicity; the vaccine produced one PR in one patient and prolonged SD in multiple patients, especially in KRAS gastrointestinal cancer mutant patients [155].

Similarly, a first-in-human trial of the LV305 vaccine, a vaccine using DCs transduced with a lentivirus expressing the NY-ESO-1 antigen, demonstrated a favourable safety profile with grade 1/2 event such as fatigue (49%), injection (46%) and myalgia (21%); induction of anti-NY-ESO-1-specific CD4+ and CD8+ responses were observed, with a DCR of 56.4% in all patients and 62% in sarcoma patients [159].

2.4.6 Oncolytic virus vaccines

Oncolytic viruses are a particular category of viruses that have the characteristic of infecting both healthy and tumour cells, but of selectively replicating only in the latter. They therefore kill tumour cells, additionally inducing activation of innate and adaptive immune responses through immunogenic tumour cell death [156]. As for viral vectors, they also offer the possibility to express cytotoxic or immunomodulatory molecules. The herpes virus vaccine called T-VEC, engineered to selectively replicate in tumour cells and to secrete GM-CSF, has been approved by the FDA for intratumoural administration for stage IIIB/C-IV melanoma based on the phase 3 OPTiM trial [51, 157], as mentioned above (see Section 2.2.1). A recently reported series of off-trial uses of T-VEC in early advanced melanoma (stages IIIB/C-IVM1a) showed a CR rate of 61.5% and a PR rate of 26.9, with a DCR of 92.3% [158].

T-VEC is also being tested in other malignancies. In HNSCC, T-VEC was used in combination with standard chemoradiation for untreated unresectable stage III/IV disease in a phase 1/2 trial. At a median follow-up of 29 months, PFS was 76%, very importantly demonstrating the safety and feasibility of this combination approach [159]. The initial design of the phase 3 trial was subsequently modified in view of the introduction of pembrolizumab in the standard of care management of HNSCC and was redesigned as a phase 1b trial randomising patients to pembrolizumab with or without T-VEC delivered to involved cervical nodes (MASTERKEY-232, NCT2626000). This trial showed a manageable safety profile, with however 24/36 (66.7%) patients experiencing serious adverse events, including one vaccine-related death. The overall response rate was 16.7%, the majority of which was in patients with PD-L1-positive tumours, and the DCR was 38.9% (again mostly in PD-L1-positive tumours) [160].

2.5 Vaccine adjuvants

Vaccination "per se" can activate antigen-specific T cells. However, when the antigen is in the form of peptides, proteins or even tumour cells, they are usually not strong enough to induce an immune response that leads to tumour eradication. The reason for this is that these antigens come without pathogen-associated molecular pattern (PAMPs) that can be recognised by innate immune cells. Most cancer vaccines are therefore combined with adjuvants, which, in addition to eliciting an innate immune response, have the role of protecting the antigen from degradation, ensuring prolonged release and promoting antigen uptake by DCs. The efficiency and choice of the adjuvant heavily influences the vaccine efficacy.

Adjuvants that act as delivery systems are classified into virosomes, liposomes, the saponin QS-21, mineral salts and the water-in-oil emulsion Montanide (an incomplete Freund's adjuvant analogue). Montanide is used in many trials of peptide vaccines and is generally well tolerated [61]. Aluminium is mostly used for antiviral vaccines such as the HPV vaccine as it promotes humoral rather than cellular responses [61]. Immunostimulatory complexes (ISCOMs) are ring-like structures containing lipids and saponin and can incorporate the antigen for optimal presentation for DCs. GM-CSF, which is employed to recruit and activate DCs at the injection site, is also being used in a large number of trials [61].

Innate immune stimulatory adjuvants are dominated by TLR ligands, but STING ligands, C-type lectin receptor (CLR) ligands and RIG-like receptor (RLR) ligands are also being tested [161]. TLR ligands induce a strong activation of DCs, and currently tested molecules include agonists to TLR2, TRL3 (e.g. the dsRNA analogue poly-ICLC), TLR7/8 (e.g. imiquimod) and TLR9 (e.g. the bacterial dinucleotide DNA CpGs). Many trials using CpGs have demonstrated its potential to improve T-cell responses, but it is now difficult to have access to it. Imiquimod is approved for the treatment of basal cell carcinoma and is used in combination with vaccines in several trials [61]. The TLR4 agonist glucopyranosyl lipid A (GLA) is currently used as adjuvants in peptide vaccines, such as with the NY-ESO-1 antigen [166]. Use of poly-ICLC is increasing, mostly for GBM vaccine trials, at it has proposed to favour T-cell homing to the brain [162].

Although many of the above-mentioned adjuvants are promising, the fear that using them alone would not induce strong enough immune response has led to development of combination strategies. Montanide is commonly used to protect the antigen in combination with a TLR ligand to promote inflammation. However, combining several immunostimulatory adjuvants such as two or more TLR ligands is being tested. Many more combination can be envisaged as long as safety is preserved.

2.6 Vaccine combinations

Vaccines, when efficiently designed, have the ability to induce strong T-cell responses. However, this does not imply that these T cells will be allowed to function at the tumour site, for several reasons. These include, among others, the immunosuppressive tumour microenvironment and the induction of immune checkpoint molecules on T cells. In an attempt to target these mechanisms, many combinations of vaccines with other immunotherapeutic strategies are currently in development. Checkpoint inhibitors, agonist antibodies and immunostimulatory cytokines can increase tumour cell immune destruction. Moreover, combining with radiotherapy, hormonotherapy and chemotherapy may also be synergistic.

2.6.1 Vaccines + checkpoint inhibitors

2.6.1.1 Vaccine + anti-CTLA-4 antibodies

CTLA-4 is expressed on T cells after activation as part of the normal regulation process of immune responses. However, in the case of antitumour responses, function of T cells need to be sustained, which is prevented by CTLA-4 expression [163]. To prevent that, two anti-CTLA-4 monoclonal antibodies, ipilimumab and tremelimumab, are currently in various stages of clinical development in combination with vaccines.

As examples, the PROSTVAC vaccine was tested with ipilimumab in mCRPC in a phase 1 escalation clinical trial. As a result, 14 of the 24 chemotherapy-naïve patients had reduction in PSA. Median OS was 31.3 months, which was longer than PROSTVAC alone [164]. This vaccine is currently being tested in combination with other checkpoint inhibitors (NCT2506114, NCT02933255, and NCT03532217).

GVAX was studied in combination with ipilimumab in 28 mCRPC patients in a phase 1 trial. Around 39% grade 3/4 irAEs were seen (most common: hypophysitis, alveolitis and hepatitis). About 25% had >50% decline in PSA, while 53.5% had SD radiologically [165]. GVAX has also been combined with ipilimumab in 30 pancreatic adenocarcinoma patients, versus ipilimumab alone [166]. The combination arm showed that three patients had extended SD and seven patients had a reduction in their tumour marker.

2.6.1.2 Vaccines + PD-1/PD-L1 inhibitors

PD-1 is a protein expressed on T cells, some B cells and NK cells, and binding of its ligands PD-L1 and PD-L2 results in cell inhibition [163]. PD1 ligands can be expressed not only by tumour cells but also by other cells of the tumour microenvironment, and PD-L1 has been shown to be induced as a result of T-cell activity [167]. The blocking of this interaction is being tested with the aim to allow prolonged T-cell activity to take place, and several anti-PD1 (pembrolizumab and nivolumab, among others) and anti-PD-L1 (atezolizumab, avelumab and durvalumab) antibodies have been developed.

Among others, combination of nivolumab with a multipeptide vaccine has been evaluated for the adjuvant treatment of high-risk melanoma. Results were promising, showing a median PFS of 47.1 months compared to historical median of 5–7.2 months with other approaches [168].

Pembrolizumab has been combined with a DNA vaccine encoding PAP in mCRPC patients. PSA responses were more important in the cohort receiving concurrent than sequential treatment. PSA declines were associated with the development of PAP-specific Th1-biased T-cell immunity and $CD8^+$ T-cell infiltration in metastatic tumour biopsy specimens. No confirmed CR or PR was observed; however, 4/5 patients treated concurrently had measurable decreases in tumour volume at 12 weeks [169].

A multitude of studies are currently testing vaccines combinations with checkpoint inhibitors for different malignancies.

2.6.2 Vaccines + tyrosine kinase inhibitors

Tyrosine kinase inhibitors (TKIs) have been used for the treatment of several solid tumours and haematological malignancies. There is preclinical and clinical data proposing that TKIs have an “off-target” effect on immune cells that restraint and/or intensify the antitumour response [170].

A phase 3 trial evaluating the combination of sunitinib with a modified vaccinia Ankara-based vaccine encoding the tumour-associated antigen 5T4 (MVA-5T4) was not able to demonstrate benefit in OS, although patients with good-risk tumours responded better to the combination [171].

Based on the positive results of a phase 3 trial evaluating the epidermal growth factor (EGF) vaccine CIMAvax-EGF as switch maintenance therapy versus placebo for previously chemo-treated advanced NSCLC patients [172], a phase 1b study evaluating the CIMAvax-EGF vaccine in combination with *EGFR* TKI in *EGFR*-mutated NSCLC tumours (EPICAL trial) is currently ongoing (NCT03623750).

2.6.3 Vaccines + endocrine treatment

Endocrine treatment is important in hormonally driven tumours like prostate and breast cancer. Patients treated with letrozole, an aromatase inhibitor used for the adjuvant treatment of hormone-responsive breast cancer, were found to have less Tregs in the tumour microenvironment [172]. In addition, androgen deprivation therapy in prostate cancer patients generates an immunostimulatory microenvironment increasing the number of effector T cells [173, 174].

A post hoc analysis of a phase 3 randomised trial of the Sialyl Tn-KLH vaccine in women with metastatic breast cancer indicated an improved clinical outcome with the addition of concomitant endocrine therapy, with prolonged time to progression and OS [175]. The order of sequential treatment seemed to be important; a combination crossover study of nilutamide with a PSA-encoding poxvirus-based vaccine in non-metastatic CRPC suggested improved OS when the vaccine was administered before the hormonotherapy [176].

These combinations are attractive therapy options for hormonosensitive cancers because vaccines are minimally toxic and can easily be incorporated into standard of care regimens.

2.6.4 Vaccines + chemotherapy

Chemotherapy agents are known to induce reduction in both $CD4^+$ and $CD8^+$ T cells, however still allowing for immune responses to occur [177]. Several chemotherapeutic agents such as gemcitabine, taxanes, topoisomerase inhibitors, platinum compounds and 5-FU have been shown to produce immunomodulatory effects [177, 178].

The OPT-822 vaccine in combination with cyclophosphamide was tested in a phase 2/3 study in metastatic breast cancer versus cyclophosphamide plus placebo. The vaccination arm failed to show a PFS or interim OS benefit in the overall study population; however, they were significantly improved in the 50% of patients that developed an immune response to the vaccination [179].

IMA950 is a multipeptide GBM-specific vaccine composed of tumour-associated MHC class I- and II-restricted peptides [179]. The vaccine has been combined with standard chemoradiotherapy and adjuvant temozolomide in patients with newly diagnosed GBM in two reported trials. A phase 1 study of IMA950 adjuvanted with GM-CSF showed that the primary immunogenicity endpoint of observing multi-antigen responses in at least 30% of patients was reached. PFS was 74% at 6 months and 31% at 9 months [180]. The second clinical trial was a phase 1/2 trial of the IMA950 vaccine adjuvanted with poly-ICLC in high-grade gliomas; CD8 T-cell responses to a single or multiple peptides were observed in 63.2% and 36.8% of patients, respectively, while median OS was 19 months, comparing favourably to classical chemoradiation results [181]. A phase 1/2 trial evaluating the combination of the IMA950 vaccine with pembrolizumab in recurrent GBM is currently ongoing (NCT03665545).

2.6.5 Vaccines + radiotherapy

The concept of synergy between vaccines and radiotherapy attracts growing interest in cancer therapy. One of the hypotheses to explain this is that radiation can not only elicit a tumour-specific immune response locally but also at distant sites, therefore acting as an in situ vaccine, eliciting both local and systemic responses [182]. Many trials have tested and are currently testing vaccines and radiotherapy, and hope is that they will provide important information on how to optimise cancer vaccines.

3. Conclusions

Vaccine immunotherapy currently shows a prolific activity in early phase trials and an expanding pipeline, with however few successes in late phase trials, despite encouraging or promising early results, resulting in a limited number of approved drugs with modest therapeutic benefit. Furthermore, there have been therapeutic vaccine studies reported in the early or mid-2000s, without further translation or progression to later trial phases.

As our understanding of the potential of immunotherapy expands so does the list of research questions that will need to be answered before this approach can be translated for effective clinical use. Can the thus far limited success, reflected by the very few approved drugs, be attributed to suboptimal or inadequate trial design? What is the optimal endpoint for vaccine trials? How long would we need to treat patients with immune modulatory therapies? What is the best combination of approaches? What is the optimal sequence strategy?

It is evident that, in order to proceed in the next stage of therapeutic vaccine development, paradigm changes ought to probably be made towards more optimal utilisation of resources and therapeutic potential. We need a clearly defined clinical readout for therapeutic response, and we need a blueprint for successful translation. We might need to consider that the concept of using vaccines in stage IV disease is not the correct way forward, but rather bringing vaccines in earlier disease stages and developing adjuvant or maintenance strategies. In this context, OS might not be the correct endpoint to use, but disease-free or relapse-free survival might be more appropriate. Our understanding of the evolution of immune escape is still incomplete, and additional work must be done to identify those patients who will benefit most from immunotherapy and to develop novel strategies.

Author details

Carmen Murias Henriquez[1*], Hendrik-Tobias Arkenau[1,2], Valérie Dutoit[3†] and Anna Patrikidou[1,2†]

1 Drug Development Unit, Sarah Cannon Research Institute, UK

2 Drug Development Unit, Sarah Cannon Research Institute UK and UCL Cancer Institute, UK

3 Laboratory of Tumour Immunology, Translational Research Centre in Oncohaematology, University of Geneva, Geneva, Switzerland

*Address all correspondence to: carmen.murias@hcahealthcare.co.uk

† Both are co-senior authors of equal contribution.

IntechOpen

© 2019 The Author(s). Licensee IntechOpen. This chapter is distributed under the terms of the Creative Commons Attribution License (http://creativecommons.org/licenses/by/3.0), which permits unrestricted use, distribution, and reproduction in any medium, provided the original work is properly cited.

References

[1] Siegel RL, Miller KD, Jemal A. Cancer statistics, 2018. CA: A Cancer Journal for Clinicians. 2018;**68**(1):7-30

[2] Bray F et al. Global cancer statistics 2018: GLOBOCAN estimates of incidence and mortality worldwide for 36 cancers in 185 countries. CA: A Cancer Journal for Clinicians. 2018;**68**(6):394-424

[3] Global Cancer Observatory. Available from: http://gco.iarc.fr/

[4] Fridman WH et al. The immune contexture in cancer prognosis and treatment. Nature Reviews. Clinical Oncology. 2017;**14**(12):717-734

[5] Couzin-Frankel J. Breakthrough of the year 2013. Cancer Immunotherapy. Science. 2013;**342**(6165):1432-1433

[6] Castellarin M et al. Driving cars to the clinic for solid tumors. Gene Therapy. 2018;**25**(3):165-175

[7] Pettitt D et al. CAR-T cells: A systematic review and mixed methods analysis of the clinical trials landscape. Molecular Therapy. 2018;**26**(2):342-353

[8] Morales A, Eidinger D, Bruce AW. Intracavitary Bacillus Calmette-Guerin in the treatment of superficial bladder tumors. The Journal of Urology. 1976;**116**(2):180-183

[9] Conry RM et al. Talimogene laherparepvec: First in class oncolytic virotherapy. Human Vaccines & Immunotherapeutics. 2018;**14**(4):839-846

[10] Kantoff PW et al. Sipuleucel-T immunotherapy for castration-resistant prostate cancer. New England Journal of Medicine. 2010;**363**(5):411-422

[11] Woo SR, Corrales L, Gajewski TF. Innate immune recognition of cancer. Annual Review of Immunology. 2015;**33**:445-474

[12] Largeot A et al. The B-side of cancer immunity: The underrated tune. Cell. 2019;**8**(5):449

[13] Steinman RM. Decisions about dendritic cells: Past, present, and future. Annual Review of Immunology. 2012;**30**:1-22

[14] Zhu J, Paul WE. CD4 T cells: Fates, functions, and faults. Blood. 2008;**112**(5):1557-1569

[15] GabrilovichDI,Ostrand-RosenbergS, Bronte V. Coordinated regulation of myeloid cells by tumours. Nature Reviews Immunology. 2012;**12**:253

[16] Balkwill F, Charles KA, Mantovani A. Smoldering and polarized inflammation in the initiation and promotion of malignant disease. Cancer Cell. 2005;**7**(3):211-217

[17] Mittal D et al. New insights into cancer immunoediting and its three component phases—Elimination, equilibrium and escape. Current Opinion in Immunology. 2014;**27**:16-25

[18] Donnou S et al. Murine models of B-cell lymphomas: Promising tools for designing cancer therapies. Advances in Hematology. 2012;**2012**:13

[19] Boshoff C, Weiss R. AIDS-related malignancies. Nature Reviews Cancer. 2002;**2**(5):373-382

[20] Weaver JL. Establishing the carcinogenic risk of immunomodulatory drugs. Toxicologic Pathology. 2012;**40**(2):267-271

[21] Dunn GP et al. Cancer immunoediting: From immunosurveillance to tumor escape. Nature Immunology. 2002;**3**(11):991-998

[22] Yuan J et al. Integrated NY-ESO-1 antibody and $CD8^+$ T-cell responses

correlate with clinical benefit in advanced melanoma patients treated with ipilimumab. Proceedings of the National Academy of Sciences. 2011;**108**(40):16723-16728

[23] Ostroumov D et al. CD4 and CD8 T lymphocyte interplay in controlling tumor growth. Cellular and Molecular Life Sciences. 2018;**75**(4):689-713

[24] Koebel CM et al. Adaptive immunity maintains occult cancer in an equilibrium state. Nature. 2007;**450**(7171):903-907

[25] Schreiber RD, Old LJ, Smyth MJ. Cancer immunoediting: Integrating immunity's roles in cancer suppression and promotion. Science. 2011;**331**(6024):1565-1570

[26] Vesely MD et al. Natural innate and adaptive immunity to cancer. Annual Review of Immunology. 2011;**29**(1):235-271

[27] Gajewski TF et al. Molecular profiling to identify relevant immune resistance mechanisms in the tumor microenvironment. Current Opinion in Immunology. 2011;**23**(2):286-292

[28] Miller JF, Sadelain M. The journey from discoveries in fundamental immunology to cancer immunotherapy. Cancer Cell. 2015;**27**(4):439-449

[29] Adams JL et al. Big opportunities for small molecules in immuno-oncology. Nature Reviews Drug Discovery. 2015;**14**:603

[30] Rosenberg SA, Restifo NP. Adoptive cell transfer as personalized immunotherapy for human cancer. Science. 2015;**348**(6230):62-68

[31] Ribas A, Wolchok JD. Cancer immunotherapy using checkpoint blockade. Science. 2018;**359**(6382):1350-1355

[32] Hollingsworth RE, Jansen K. Turning the corner on therapeutic cancer vaccines. npj Vaccines. 2019;**4**(1):7

[33] Keating GM. Bevacizumab: A review of its use in advanced cancer. Drugs. 2014;**74**(16):1891-1925

[34] Weiner LM, Dhodapkar MV, Ferrone S. Monoclonal antibodies for cancer immunotherapy. The Lancet. 2009;**373**(9668):1033-1040

[35] Berraondo P et al. Cytokines in clinical cancer immunotherapy. British Journal of Cancer. 2019;**120**(1):6-15

[36] Mortara L et al. Anti-cancer therapies employing IL-2 cytokine tumor targeting: Contribution of innate, adaptive and immunosuppressive cells in the anti-tumor efficacy. Frontiers in Immunology. 2018;**9**:2905-2915

[37] Mishra P, Nayak B, Dey RK. PEGylation in anti-cancer therapy: An overview. Asian Journal of Pharmaceutical Sciences. 2016;**11**(3):337-348

[38] Barroso-Sousa R, Ott PA. Transformation of old concepts for a new era of cancer immunotherapy: Cytokine therapy and cancer vaccines as combination partners of PD1/PD-L1 inhibitors. Current Oncology Reports. 2018;**20**(12):1

[39] Uy GL, Rettig MP, Cashen AF. Plerixafor, a CXCR4 antagonist for the mobilization of hematopoietic stem cells. Expert Opinion on Biological Therapy. 2008;**8**(11):1797-1804

[40] Zhu MMT, Dancsok AR, Nielsen TO. Indoleamine dioxygenase inhibitors: Clinical rationale and current development. Current Oncology Reports. 2019;**21**(1):2

[41] Yap TA et al. First-in-human study of KHK2455, a long-acting, potent and selective indoleamine 2,3-dioxygenase 1 (IDO-1) inhibitor, in combination

with mogamulizumab (Moga), an anti-CCR4 monoclonal antibody, in patients (pts) with advanced solid tumors. Journal of Clinical Oncology. 2018;**36**(15_suppl):3040-3040

[42] Leone RD, Emens LA. Targeting adenosine for cancer immunotherapy. Journal for Immunotherapy of Cancer. 2018;**6**(1):57

[43] Rohaan MW et al. Adoptive transfer of tumor-infiltrating lymphocytes in melanoma: A viable treatment option. Journal for Immunotherapy of Cancer. 2018;**6**(1):102

[44] Bonini C, Mondino A. Adoptive T-cell therapy for cancer: The era of engineered T cells. European Journal of Immunology. 2015;**45**(9):2457-2469

[45] Sadelain M, Brentjens R, Riviere I. The basic principles of chimeric antigen receptor design. Cancer Discovery. 2013;**3**(4):388-398

[46] Brown CE, Mackall CL. CAR T cell therapy: Inroads to response and resistance. Nature Reviews Immunology. 2019;**19**(2):73-74

[47] Gomes C, Wong RJ, Gish RG. Global perspective on hepatitis B virus infections in the era of effective vaccines. Clinics in Liver Disease. 2019;**23**(3):383-399

[48] Stanley M. Tumour virus vaccines: Hepatitis B virus and human papillomavirus. Philosophical Transactions of the Royal Society B: Biological Sciences. 2017;**372**(1732):20160268

[49] Lamm DL et al. A randomized trial of intravesical doxorubicin and immunotherapy with Bacille Calmette-Guérin for transitional-cell carcinoma of the bladder. New England Journal of Medicine. 1991;**325**(17):1205-1209

[50] Huber ML et al. Interdisciplinary critique of Sipuleucel-T as immunotherapy in castration-resistant prostate cancer. JNCI: Journal of the National Cancer Institute. 2012;**104**(4):273-279

[51] Andtbacka RHI et al. Talimogene laherparepvec improves durable response rate in patients with advanced melanoma. Journal of Clinical Oncology. 2015;**33**(25):2780-2788

[52] Ribas A et al. Determinant spreading and tumor responses after peptide-based cancer immunotherapy. Trends in Immunology. 2003;**24**(2):58-61

[53] van der Bruggen P et al. A gene encoding an antigen recognized by cytolytic T lymphocytes on a human melanoma. Science. 1991;**254**(5038):1643-1647

[54] Coulie PG et al. Tumour antigens recognized by T lymphocytes: At the core of cancer immunotherapy. Nature Reviews Cancer. 2014;**14**(2):135-146

[55] Fratta E et al. The biology of cancer testis antigens: Putative function, regulation and therapeutic potential. Molecular Oncology. 2011;**5**(2):164-182

[56] Wei X et al. Cancer-testis antigen peptide vaccine for cancer immunotherapy: Progress and prospects. Translational Oncology. 2019;**12**(5):733-738

[57] Bezu L et al. Trial watch: Peptide-based vaccines in anticancer therapy. OncoImmunology. 2018;**7**(12):e1511506

[58] Vigneron N. Human tumor antigens and cancer immunotherapy. BioMed Research International. 2015;**2015**:17

[59] Castle JC et al. Exploiting the mutanome for tumor vaccination. Cancer Research. 2012;**72**(5):1081-1091

[60] Finn OJ, Rammensee H-G. Is it possible to develop cancer vaccines

to neoantigens, what are the major challenges, and how can these be overcome?: Neoantigens: Nothing new in spite of the name. Cold Spring Harbor Perspectives in Biology. 2018;**10**(11):a028829-a028836

[61] Gouttefangeas C, Rammensee H-G. Personalized cancer vaccines: Adjuvants are important, too. Cancer Immunology, Immunotherapy. 2018;**67**(12):1911-1918

[62] Khong H, Overwijk WW. Adjuvants for peptide-based cancer vaccines. Journal for Immunotherapy of Cancer. 2016;**4**(1):56

[63] Kirkwood JM et al. Immunogenicity and antitumor effects of vaccination with peptide vaccine+/−granulocyte-monocyte colony-stimulating factor and/or IFN-alpha2b in advanced metastatic melanoma: Eastern Cooperative Oncology Group Phase II Trial E1696. Clinical Cancer Research. 2009;**15**(4):1443-1451

[64] Slingluff CL et al. A randomized phase II trial of multiepitope vaccination with melanoma peptides for cytotoxic T cells and helper T cells for patients with metastatic melanoma (E1602). Clinical Cancer Research. 2013;**19**(15):4228-4238

[65] Pollack IF et al. Antigen-specific immune responses and clinical outcome after vaccination with glioma-associated antigen peptides and polyinosinic-polycytidylic acid stabilized by lysine and carboxymethylcellulose in children with newly diagnosed malignant brainstem and nonbrainstem gliomas. Journal of Clinical Oncology. 2014;**32**(19):2050-2058

[66] Parmiani G et al. Cancer immunotherapy with peptide-based vaccines: What have we achieved? Where are we going? JNCI: Journal of the National Cancer Institute. 2002;**94**(11):805-818

[67] Guo C et al. Therapeutic cancer vaccines: Past, present, and future. Advances in Cancer Research. 2013;**119**:421-475

[68] Antony PA et al. $CD8^+$ T cell immunity against a tumor/self-antigen is augmented by $CD4^+$ T helper cells and hindered by naturally occurring T regulatory cells. The Journal of Immunology. 2005;**174**(5):2591-2601

[69] van der Burg SH. Correlates of immune and clinical activity of novel cancer vaccines. Seminars in Immunology. 2018;**39**:119-136

[70] Jr CLS et al. Immunologic and clinical outcomes of vaccination with a multiepitope melanoma peptide vaccine plus low-dose interleukin-2 administered either concurrently or on a delayed schedule. Journal of Clinical Oncology. 2004;**22**(22):4474-4485

[71] Slingluff CL et al. Immunologic and clinical outcomes of a randomized phase II trial of two multipeptide vaccines for melanoma in the adjuvant setting. Clinical Cancer Research. 2007;**13**(21):6386-6395

[72] Jr CLS et al. Randomized multicenter trial of the effects of melanoma-associated helper peptides and cyclophosphamide on the immunogenicity of a multipeptide melanoma vaccine. Journal of Clinical Oncology. 2011;**29**(21):2924-2932

[73] Hos BJ et al. Approaches to improve chemically defined synthetic peptide vaccines. Frontiers in Immunology. 2018;**9**:884-891

[74] Swee LK et al. Sortase-mediated modification of αDEC205 affords optimization of antigen presentation and immunization against a set of viral epitopes. Proceedings of the National Academy of Sciences. 2013;**110**(4):1428-1433

[75] Rahimian S et al. Polymeric nanoparticles for co-delivery of synthetic long peptide antigen and poly IC as therapeutic cancer vaccine formulation. Journal of Controlled Release. 2015;**203**:16-22

[76] Varypataki EM et al. Synthetic long peptide-based vaccine formulations for induction of cell mediated immunity: A comparative study of cationic liposomes and PLGA nanoparticles. Journal of Controlled Release. 2016;**226**:98-106

[77] Walter S et al. Multipeptide immune response to cancer vaccine IMA901 after single-dose cyclophosphamide associates with longer patient survival. Nature Medicine. 2012;**18**(8):1254-1261

[78] Rini BI et al. IMA901, a multipeptide cancer vaccine, plus sunitinib versus sunitinib alone, as first-line therapy for advanced or metastatic renal cell carcinoma (IMPRINT): A multicentre, open-label, randomised, controlled, phase 3 trial. The Lancet Oncology. 2016;**17**(11):1599-1611

[79] Hipp MM et al. Sorafenib, but not sunitinib, affects function of dendritic cells and induction of primary immune responses. Blood. 2008;**111**(12):5610-5620

[80] Finke JH et al. Sunitinib reverses Type-1 immune suppression and decreases T-regulatory cells in renal cell carcinoma patients. Clinical Cancer Research. 2008;**14**(20):6674-6682

[81] Ko JS et al. Sunitinib mediates reversal of myeloid-derived suppressor cell accumulation in renal cell carcinoma patients. Clinical Cancer Research. 2009;**15**(6):2148-2157

[82] Ott PA et al. An immunogenic personal neoantigen vaccine for patients with melanoma. Nature. 2017;**547**:217

[83] Sahin U et al. Personalized RNA mutanome vaccines mobilize poly-specific therapeutic immunity against cancer. Nature. 2017;**547**:222

[84] Kimura T et al. MUC1 vaccine for individuals with advanced adenoma of the colon: A cancer immunoprevention feasibility study. Cancer Prevention Research. 2012;**6**(1):18-26

[85] Clifton GT et al. Clinical development of the E75 vaccine in breast cancer. Breast Care. 2016;**11**(2):116-121

[86] Mittendorf EA et al. Final report of the phase I/II clinical trial of the E75 (nelipepimut-S) vaccine with booster inoculations to prevent disease recurrence in high-risk breast cancer patients. Annals of Oncology. 2014;**25**(9):1735-1742

[87] Pelloski CE et al. Epidermal growth factor receptor variant III status defines clinically distinct subtypes of glioblastoma. Journal of Clinical Oncology. 2007;**25**(16):2288-2294

[88] Sampson JH et al. Greater chemotherapy-induced lymphopenia enhances tumor-specific immune responses that eliminate EGFRvIII-expressing tumor cells in patients with glioblastoma. Neuro-Oncology. 2010;**13**(3):324-333

[89] Schuster J et al. A phase II, multicenter trial of rindopepimut (CDX-110) in newly diagnosed glioblastoma: The ACT III study. Neuro-Oncology. 2015;**17**(6):854-861

[90] Weller M et al. Rindopepimut with temozolomide for patients with newly diagnosed, EGFRvIII-expressing glioblastoma (ACT IV): A randomised, double-blind, international phase 3 trial. The Lancet Oncology. 2017;**18**(10):1373-1385

[91] Reardon DA et al. IMCT-08 ReACT: Long-term survival from a randomized

phase II study of rindopepimut (CDX-110) plus bevacizumab in relapsed glioblastoma. Neuro-Oncology. 2015;**17**(suppl_5):v109-v109

[92] Pizzurro GA, Barrio MM. Dendritic cell-based vaccine efficacy: Aiming for hot spots. Frontiers in Immunology. 2015;**6**:91

[93] Nestle FO et al. Vaccination of melanoma patients with peptide- or tumorlysate-pulsed dendritic cells. Nature Medicine. 1998;**4**(3):328-332

[94] Banchereau J et al. Immune and clinical responses in patients with metastatic melanoma to $CD34^+$ progenitor-derived dendritic cell vaccine. Cancer Research. 2001;**61**(17):6451-6458

[95] Palucka K, Banchereau J. Cancer immunotherapy via dendritic cells. Nature Reviews Cancer. 2012;**12**:265

[96] Fong L et al. Neoadjuvant sipuleucel-T in localized prostate cancer: Effects on immune cells within the prostate tumor microenvironment. Journal of Clinical Oncology. 2012;**30**(15_suppl):2564-2564

[97] Wierecky J et al. Immunologic and clinical responses after vaccinations with peptide-pulsed dendritic cells in metastatic renal cancer patients. Cancer Research. 2006;**66**(11):5910-5918

[98] Van Tendeloo VF et al. Induction of complete and molecular remissions in acute myeloid leukemia by Wilms' tumor 1 antigen-targeted dendritic cell vaccination. Proceedings of the National Academy of Sciences. 2010;**107**(31):13824-13829

[99] Rosenblatt J et al. Individualized vaccination of AML patients in remission is associated with induction of antileukemia immunity and prolonged remissions. Science Translational Medicine. 2016;**8**(368):368ra171-368ra171

[100] Liau LM et al. Dendritic cell vaccination in glioblastoma patients induces systemic and intracranial T-cell responses modulated by the local central nervous system tumor microenvironment. Clinical Cancer Research. 2005;**11**(15):5515-5525

[101] Prins RM et al. Gene expression profile correlates with T-cell infiltration and relative survival in glioblastoma patients vaccinated with dendritic cell immunotherapy. Clinical Cancer Research. 2011;**17**(6):1603-1615

[102] Liau LM et al. First results on survival from a large phase 3 clinical trial of an autologous dendritic cell vaccine in newly diagnosed glioblastoma. Journal of Translational Medicine. 2018;**16**(1):142

[103] Bonehill A et al. Single-step antigen loading and activation of dendritic cells by mRNA electroporation for the purpose of therapeutic vaccination in melanoma patients. Clinical Cancer Research. 2009;**15**(10):3366-3375

[104] Bonehill A et al. Enhancing the T-cell stimulatory capacity of human dendritic cells by co-electroporation with CD40L, CD70 and constitutively active TLR4 encoding mRNA. Molecular Therapy. 2008;**16**(6):1170-1180

[105] Minkis K et al. Type 2 bias of T cells expanded from the blood of melanoma patients switched to type 1 by *IL-12p70* mRNA-transfected dendritic cells. Cancer Research. 2008;**68**(22):9441-9450

[106] Breckpot K et al. Attenuated expression of A20 markedly increases the efficacy of double-stranded RNA-activated dendritic cells as an anti-cancer vaccine. The Journal of Immunology. 2009;**182**(2):860-870

[107] Yi H et al. Targeting the immunoregulator SRA/CD204 potentiates specific dendritic cell

vaccine-induced T-cell response and antitumor immunity. Cancer Research. 2011;**71**(21):6611-6620

[108] Rüttinger D et al. Adjuvant therapeutic vaccination in patients with non-small cell lung cancer made lymphopenic and reconstituted with autologous PBMC: First clinical experience and evidence of an immune response. Journal of Translational Medicine. 2007;**5**(1):43

[109] Baars A et al. Skin tests predict survival after autologous tumor cell vaccination in metastatic melanoma: Experience in 81 patients. Annals of Oncology. 2000;**11**(8):965-970

[110] Berd D et al. Immunopharmacologic analysis of an autologous, Hapten-modified human melanoma vaccine. Journal of Clinical Oncology. 2004;**22**(3):403-415

[111] Antonia SJ et al. Phase I trial of a B7-1 (CD80) gene modified autologous tumor cell vaccine in combination with systemic interleukin-2 in patients with metastatic renal cell carcinoma. The Journal of Urology. 2002;**167**(5):1995-2000

[112] Berger M et al. Phase I study with an autologous tumor cell vaccine for locally advanced or metastatic prostate cancer. Journal of Pharmacy & Pharmaceutical Sciences. 2007;**10**(2):144-152

[113] Harris JE et al. Adjuvant active specific immunotherapy for stage II and III colon cancer with an autologous tumor cell vaccine: Eastern cooperative oncology group study E5283. Journal of Clinical Oncology. 2000;**18**(1):148-148

[114] Hanna JMG. Immunotherapy with autologous tumor cell vaccines for treatment of occult disease in early stage colon cancer. Human Vaccines & Immunotherapeutics. 2012;**8**(8):1156-1160

[115] Lathuilière A, Mach N, Schneider BL. Encapsulated cellular implants for recombinant protein delivery and therapeutic modulation of the immune system. International Journal of Molecular Sciences. 2015;**16**(5):10578-10600

[116] Migliorini D et al. 531 MVX-ONCO-1: First in man, phase I clinical trial combining encapsulation cell technology and irradiated autologous tumor cells for personalized cell-based immunotherapy. Safety, feasibility and clinical outcome results. European Journal of Cancer. 2015;**51**:S114

[117] Migliorini D et al. First report of clinical responses to immunotherapy in 3 relapsing cases of chordoma after failure of standard therapies. OncoImmunology. 2017;**6**(8):e1338235

[118] Morton DL et al. Prolongation of survival in metastatic melanoma after active specific immunotherapy with a new polyvalent melanoma vaccine. Annals of Surgery. 1992;**216**(4):463-482

[119] Morton DL et al. Prolonged survival of patients receiving active immunotherapy with Canvaxin therapeutic polyvalent vaccine after complete resection of melanoma metastatic to regional lymph nodes. Annals of Surgery. 2002;**236**(4):438-448 discussion 448-9

[120] Hsueh EC et al. Prolonged survival after complete resection of disseminated melanoma and active immunotherapy with a therapeutic cancer vaccine. Journal of Clinical Oncology. 2002;**20**(23):4549-4554

[121] Sondak VK, Sabel MS, Mulé JJ. Allogeneic and autologous melanoma vaccines: Where have we been and where are we going? Clinical Cancer Research. 2006;**12**(7):2337s-2341s

[122] Ward S et al. Immunotherapeutic potential of whole tumour cells.

Cancer Immunology, Immunotherapy. 2002;**51**(7):351-357

[123] Simons JW et al. Phase I/II trial of an allogeneic cellular immunotherapy in hormone-Naïve prostate cancer. Clinical Cancer Research. 2006;**12**(11):3394-3401

[124] Small EJ et al. Granulocyte macrophage colony-stimulating factor–secreting allogeneic cellular immunotherapy for hormone-refractory prostate cancer. Clinical Cancer Research. 2007;**13**(13):3883-3891

[125] Emens LA et al. Timed sequential treatment with cyclophosphamide, doxorubicin, and an allogeneic granulocyte-macrophage colony-stimulating factor-secreting breast tumor vaccine: A chemotherapy dose-ranging factorial study of safety and immune activation. Journal of Clinical Oncology. 2009;**27**(35):5911-5918

[126] Lutz E et al. A lethally irradiated allogeneic granulocyte-macrophage colony stimulating factor-secreting tumor vaccine for pancreatic adenocarcinoma. A Phase II trial of safety, efficacy, and immune activation. Annals of Surgery. 2011;**253**(2):328-335

[127] Le DT et al. Results from a phase IIb, randomized, multicenter study of GVAX pancreas and CRS-207 compared with chemotherapy in adults with previously treated metastatic pancreatic adenocarcinoma (ECLIPSE study). Clinical Cancer Research; 24 June 2019. DOI: 10.1158/1078-0432.CCR-18-2992

[128] Nemunaitis J et al. Phase II trial of belagenpumatucel-L, a TGF-β2 antisense gene modified allogeneic tumor vaccine in advanced non small cell lung cancer (NSCLC) patients. Cancer Gene Therapy. 2009;**16**:620

[129] Nemunaitis J et al. Phase II study of belagenpumatucel-L, a transforming growth factor beta-2 antisense gene-modified allogeneic tumor cell vaccine in non-small-cell lung cancer. Journal of Clinical Oncology. 2006;**24**(29):4721-4730

[130] Giaccone G et al. A phase III study of belagenpumatucel-L, an allogeneic tumour cell vaccine, as maintenance therapy for non-small cell lung cancer. European Journal of Cancer. 2015;**51**(16):2321-2329

[131] Bendandi M et al. Complete molecular remissions induced by patient-specific vaccination plus granulocyte-monocyte colony-stimulating factor against lymphoma. Nature Medicine. 1999;**5**(10):1171-1177

[132] Schuster SJ et al. Vaccination with patient-specific tumor-derived antigen in first remission improves disease-free survival in follicular lymphoma. Journal of Clinical Oncology. 2011;**29**(20):2787-2794

[133] Levy R et al. Active idiotypic vaccination versus control immunotherapy for follicular lymphoma. Journal of Clinical Oncology. 2014;**32**(17):1797-1803

[134] Levy R et al. Results of a Phase 3 trial evaluating safety and efficacy of specific immunotherapy, recombinant idiotype (Id) conjugated to KLH (Id-KLH) with GM-CSF, compared to non-specific immunotherapy, KLH with GM-CSF, in patients with follicular non-Hodgkin's lymphoma (fNHL). Cancer Research. 2008;**68**(9 Supplement):LB-204

[135] Link CJ Jr et al. Eliciting hyperacute xenograft response to treat human cancer: Alpha(1,3) galactosyltransferase gene therapy. Anticancer Research. 1998;**18**(4A):2301-2308

[136] Rossi GR et al. Effective treatment of preexisting melanoma with whole cell vaccines expressing

alpha(1,3)-galactosyl epitopes. Cancer Research. 2005;**65**(22):10555-10561

[137] Hardacre JM et al. Addition of algenpantucel-L immunotherapy to standard adjuvant therapy for pancreatic cancer: A phase 2 study. Journal of Gastrointestinal Surgery. 2013;**17**(1):94-101

[138] Hemstreet GP 3rd et al. Cellular immunotherapy study of prostate cancer patients and resulting IgG responses to peptide epitopes predicted from prostate tumor-associated autoantigens. Journal of Immunotherapy. 2013;**36**(1):57-65

[139] Graner MW, Bigner DD. Chaperone proteins and brain tumors: Potential targets and possible therapeutics. Neuro-Oncology. 2005;7(3):260-278

[140] Bloch O et al. Heat-shock protein peptide complex-96 vaccination for recurrent glioblastoma: A phase II, single-arm trial. Neuro-Oncology. 2014;**16**(2):274-279

[141] Bloch O et al. Autologous heat shock protein peptide vaccination for newly diagnosed glioblastoma: Impact of peripheral PD-L1 expression on response to therapy. Clinical Cancer Research. 2017;**23**(14):3575-3584

[142] Bloch O et al. ATIM-14. Alliance A071101: A phase II randomized trial comparing the efficacy of heat shock protein peptide complex-96 (HSPPC-96) vaccine given with bevacizumab versus bevacizumab alone in the treatment of surgically resectable recurrent glioblastoma. Neuro-Oncology. 2017;**19**(suppl_6):vi29-vi29

[143] Shevtsov M, Multhoff G. Heat shock protein–peptide and HSP-based immunotherapies for the treatment of cancer. Frontiers in Immunology. 2016;7:171-177

[144] Larocca C, Schlom J. Viral vector-based therapeutic cancer vaccines. Cancer Journal. 2011;**17**(5):359-371

[145] Harrop R, John J, Carroll MW. Recombinant viral vectors: Cancer vaccines. Advanced Drug Delivery Reviews. 2006;**58**(8):931-947

[146] Gulley JL et al. Results of PROSPECT: A randomized phase 3 trial of PROSTVAC-V/F (PRO) in men with asymptomatic or minimally symptomatic metastatic, castration-resistant prostate cancer. Journal of Clinical Oncology. 2018;**36**(15_suppl):5006-5006

[147] Kantoff PW et al. Overall survival analysis of a phase II randomized controlled trial of a poxviral-based PSA-targeted immunotherapy in metastatic castration-resistant prostate cancer. Journal of Clinical Oncology. 2010;**28**(7):1099-1105

[148] Gulley JL et al. Immunologic and prognostic factors associated with overall survival employing a poxviral-based PSA vaccine in metastatic castrate-resistant prostate cancer. Cancer Immunology, Immunotherapy. 2010;**59**(5):663-674

[149] Gulley JL et al. Immune impact induced by PROSTVAC (PSA-TRICOM), a therapeutic vaccine for prostate cancer. Cancer Immunology Research. 2014;**2**(2):133-141

[150] Mohebtash M et al. A pilot study of MUC-1/CEA/TRICOM poxviral-based vaccine in patients with metastatic breast and ovarian cancer. Clinical Cancer Research. 2011;**17**(22):7164-7173

[151] Gulley JL et al. Pilot study of vaccination with recombinant CEA-MUC-1-TRICOM Poxviral-based vaccines in patients with metastatic carcinoma. Clinical Cancer Research. 2008;**14**(10):3060-3069

[152] Duggan MC et al. A phase I study of recombinant (r) vaccinia-CEA(6D)-TRICOM and rFowlpox-CEA(6D)-TRICOM vaccines with GM-CSF and IFN-α-2b in patients with CEA-expressing carcinomas. Cancer Immunology, Immunotherapy. 2016;**65**(11):1353-1364

[153] Lou E et al. A phase II study of active immunotherapy with PANVAC™ or autologous, cultured dendritic cells infected with PANVAC™ after complete resection of hepatic metastases of colorectal carcinoma. Clinical Colorectal Cancer. 2006;**5**(5):368-371

[154] Heery CR et al. Phase I study of a poxviral TRICOM-based vaccine directed against the transcription factor brachyury. Clinical Cancer Research. 2017;**23**(22):6833-6845

[155] Gatti-Mays ME et al. A phase 1 dose escalation trial of BN-CV301, a recombinant poxviral vaccine targeting MUC1 and CEA with costimulatory molecules. Clinical Cancer Research. **25**(16):4933-4944

[156] Russell L et al. Oncolytic viruses: Priming time for cancer immunotherapy. BioDrugs. 2019. https://doi.org/10.1007/s40259-019-00367-0

[157] Andtbacka RHI et al. Final analyses of OPTiM: A randomized phase III trial of talimogene laherparepvec versus granulocyte-macrophage colony-stimulating factor in unresectable stage III–IV melanoma. Journal for Immunotherapy of Cancer. 2019;**7**(1):145

[158] Franke V et al. High response rates for T-VEC in early metastatic melanoma (stage IIIB/C-IVM1a). International Journal of Cancer. 2019;**145**(4):974-978

[159] Harrington KJ et al. Phase I/II study of oncolytic HSV GM-CSF in combination with radiotherapy and cisplatin in untreated stage III/IV squamous cell cancer of the head and neck. Clinical Cancer Research. 2010;**16**(15):4005-4015

[160] Harrington KJ et al. Safety and preliminary efficacy of talimogene laherparepvec (T-VEC) in combination (combo) with pembrobrolizumab (Pembro) in patients (pts) with recurrent or metastatic squamous cell carcinoma of the head and neck (R/M HNSCC): A multicenter, phase 1b study (MASTERKEY-232). Journal of Clinical Oncology. 2018;**36**(15_suppl):6036-6036

[161] Temizoz B, Kuroda E, Ishii KJ. Vaccine adjuvants as potential cancer immunotherapeutics. International Immunology. 2016;**28**(7):329-338

[162] Okada H. Brain tumor immunotherapy with type-1 polarizing strategies. Annals of the New York Academy of Sciences. 2009;**1174**:18-23

[163] Pardoll DM. The blockade of immune checkpoints in cancer immunotherapy. Nature Reviews Cancer. 2012;**12**(4):252-264

[164] Madan RA et al. Ipilimumab and a poxviral vaccine targeting prostate-specific antigen in metastatic castration-resistant prostate cancer: A phase 1 dose-escalation trial. The Lancet Oncology. 2012;**13**(5):501-508

[165] van den Eertwegh AJM et al. Combined immunotherapy with granulocyte-macrophage colony-stimulating factor-transduced allogeneic prostate cancer cells and ipilimumab in patients with metastatic castration-resistant prostate cancer: A phase 1 dose-escalation trial. The Lancet Oncology. 2012;**13**(5):509-517

[166] Le DT et al. Evaluation of ipilimumab in combination with allogeneic pancreatic tumor cells transfected with a GM-CSF

gene in previously treated pancreatic cancer. Journal of Immunotherapy. 2013;**36**(7):382-389

[167] Alspach E, Lussier DM, Schreiber RD. Interferon γ and its important roles in promoting and inhibiting spontaneous and therapeutic cancer immunity. Cold Spring Harbor Perspectives in Biology. 2019;**11**(3):a028480-a028500

[168] Gibney GT et al. Safety, correlative markers, and clinical results of adjuvant nivolumab in combination with vaccine in resected high-risk metastatic melanoma. Clinical Cancer Research. 2015;**21**(4):712-720

[169] McNeel DG et al. Concurrent, but not sequential, PD-1 blockade with a DNA vaccine elicits anti-tumor responses in patients with metastatic, castration-resistant prostate cancer. Oncotarget. 2018;**9**(39):25586-25596

[170] Ott PA, Adams S. Small-molecule protein kinase inhibitors and their effects on the immune system: Implications for cancer treatment. Immunotherapy. 2011;**3**(2):213-227

[171] Amato RJ et al. Vaccination of metastatic renal cancer patients with MVA-5T4: A randomized, double-blind, placebo-controlled phase III study. Clinical Cancer Research. 2010;**16**(22):5539-5547

[172] Generali D et al. Immunomodulation of FOXP3^{+} regulatory T cells by the aromatase inhibitor letrozole in breast cancer patients. Clinical Cancer Research. 2009;**15**(3):1046-1051

[173] Mercader M et al. T cell infiltration of the prostate induced by androgen withdrawal in patients with prostate cancer. Proceedings of the National Academy of Sciences. 2001;**98**(25):14565-14570

[174] Drake CG et al. Androgen ablation mitigates tolerance to a prostate/prostate cancer-restricted antigen. Cancer Cell. 2005;**7**(3):239-249

[175] Ibrahim NK et al. Survival advantage in patients with metastatic breast cancer receiving endocrine therapy plus Sialyl Tn-KLH vaccine: Post hoc analysis of a large randomized trial. Journal of Cancer. 2013;**4**(7):577-584

[176] Madan RA et al. Analysis of overall survival in patients with nonmetastatic castration-resistant prostate cancer treated with vaccine, nilutamide, and combination therapy. Clinical Cancer Research. 2008;**14**(14):4526-4531

[177] Galluzzi L et al. Immunological effects of conventional chemotherapy and targeted anticancer agents. Cancer Cell. 2015;**28**(6):690-714

[178] Zitvogel L, Kroemer G. Anticancer immunochemotherapy using adjuvants with direct cytotoxic effects. The Journal of Clinical Investigation. 2009;**119**(8):2127-2130

[179] Dutoit V et al. Exploiting the glioblastoma peptidome to discover novel tumour-associated antigens for immunotherapy. Brain. 2012; **135**(Pt 4):1042-1054

[180] Rampling R et al. A cancer research UK first time in human phase I trial of IMA950 (novel multipeptide therapeutic vaccine) in patients with newly diagnosed glioblastoma. Clinical Cancer Research. 2016;**22**(19):4776-4785

[181] Migliorini D et al. Phase I/II trial testing safety and immunogenicity of the multipeptide IMA950/poly-ICLC vaccine in newly diagnosed adult malignant astrocytoma patients. Neuro-oncology. 2019;**21**(7):923-933

[182] Demaria S, Formenti S. Radiation as an immunological adjuvant: Current evidence on dose and fractionation. Frontiers in Oncology. 2012;**2**:153-159

Chapter 3

Mimetic Vaccines in Immuno-Oncology

Anastas Pashov and Thomas Kieber-Emmons

Abstract

While the interest in cancer vaccines is renewed by some results in vaccine-based clinical trials, the premise still suffers from the incomplete concept of a successful vaccine. Future progress may come from matching preclinical data with clinical expectations while taking a step back to understand the systems perspective. A field that benefits most from this bird's eye view is tumor immunology. For instance, the accumulation over the last three decades of clear associations of T and B cell cross-reactivity between a set of host targets of autoimmunity and microbial antigens strongly supports a pathogenic role for molecular mimicry. Mimicry on its turn invites the concept of networks of molecular interactions. The intentional and rational approach to exploit mimicry in cancer vaccine development, while littered with failure, has provided also some insight into success. Here, we visit successes and underlying rationale to lend to future development of mimetic vaccines in immune-oncology.

Keywords: vaccine, anti-idiotype, peptide, tumor associated carbohydrate antigens, carbohydrate mimetic peptide

1. Introduction

Targeting malignancies through manipulating the immune system has seen success in a variety approaches ranging from whole cell vaccination, to autologous dendritic cell based vaccines and therapeutic immune-modulation [1–5]. But a number of opportunities and challenges remain. While tumor antigen identification from sequencing the cancer genome continues to be a high priority we now know that tumor antigens arise from multiple mechanisms that include somatic mutations, translocations, and amplifications and post-translational modifications. The role of post-translational modification with tumor associated carbohydrate antigens (TACA) in the generation of novel cancer antigens is in particular an opportunity to be explored [6–9].

Characterizing and overcoming the immunosuppressive environment of the tumors has led to a focus on downstream checkpoints that regulate activated T cells, or on vaccination and T cell adoptive transfer to expand the T cell pool [10–12]. However, it is well known that cancer-signaling pathways play pivotal roles in the biologic behavior of tumor cells that creates an opportunity to rethink cancer in general [13] and rethink cancer targeting strategies with small molecules [14, 15], with monoclonal antibodies [16] and induced antibodies [17, 18]. By the same token such pathways are also involved in developing therapeutic resistance, which

IntechOpen

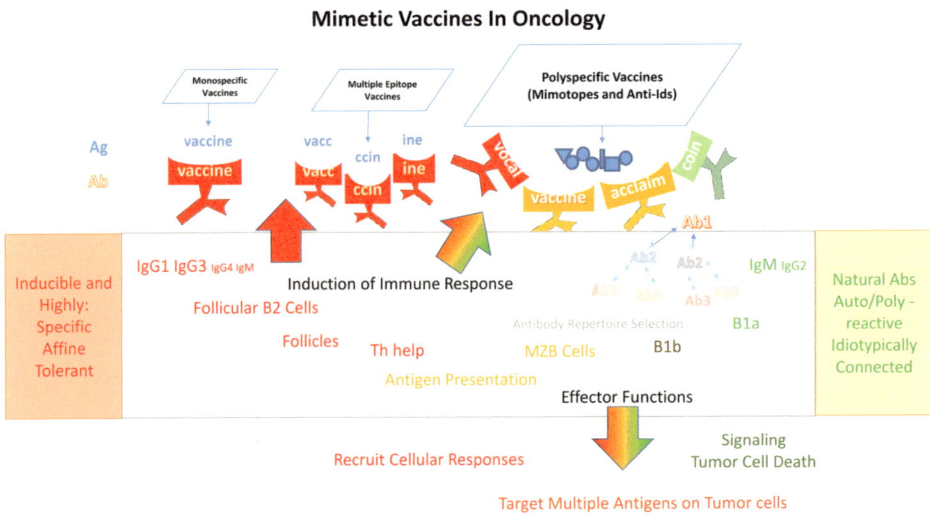

Figure 1.
The concept of mimetic vaccines in oncology. On the one end the spectrum of B cell subsets includes high affinity/specificity clones generated by somatic hypermutation in B2 follicular cells under conditions of strict tolerance to self. On the other, are the innate like B1a cells producing constitutively poly/autospecific natural antibodies. Carbohydrate specificity and anti-idiotype interactions are related more to the later compartment. Polyspecific vaccines based on carbohydrate mimotopes or idiotypes recruit B cell clones across that spectrum but their novel properties are related mostly to their capacity to elicit diversified responses from MZ and B1 cells including idiotypically connected clones. In addition, the mimotopes capture only the most salient features of the carbohydrate epitopes and induce diversified responses targeting multiple antigens (illustrated by diverse words sharing only partially the topology of the mimotope as compared to highly specific responses that match the shape of the epitope). Thus, mimetic vaccines both target polyspecific compartments of the B cell repertoire as well as they themselves function as polyspecific antigens.

requires alternative immunotherapeutic strategies. One such strategy is to develop polyclonal humoral immune responses by active immunotherapy. Itself, this concept can have multiple approaches and an orchestra of potential mechanisms that encompass a dynamic systems immunology perspective (**Figure 1**). On the one hand the effect can be pursued by formulating a platform with multiple epitopes of target antigens [19]. On the other—making use of polyspecific (pan-antigen) mimetics to target simultaneously multiple antigens on cancer cells [17, 18]. A polyclonal antibody approach would target more than two antigens on a single tumor cell, which is expected to have even higher potential. This latter idea is a part of the conceptual evolution in immune-oncology harnessing polyclonal responses to cancer cells.

2. Setting the stage: systems concepts

Systems immunology is now in focus to understand the immune system [20], especially in the context of vaccinology [21]. This perspective is ushering in a new era in vaccine development [22]. For the future, it is argued that successful approaches will depend on the elucidation of the entire network of immune signaling pathways that regulate immune responses with an eye toward integrating advances in computational and systems biology, genomics, immune monitoring, bioinformatics and machine learning [22, 23].

Systems immunology also teaches us that one antigen can substitute for another having the potential to regulate tolerance [24–28]. However, it is unclear why an immune system that is tolerant of its own self-antigens would respond to a self-antigen mimic in a vaccine. Antibodies referred to as anti-idiotypic are produced during the process of tolerization and demonstrated in tolerant animals [29, 30] and in patients [31]. These antibodies may prevent a B cell receptor from interacting with the antigen. Jerne envisioned the immune system as a web of immunoglobulin V domains constituting an idiotypic network. Inherent to the idiotype network is that antibodies recognize antibodies. Jerne thought that regulatory processes governed by idiotypic interactions could explain the generation of the various immune states that include tolerance.

An extension of the network theory was that antibodies, by virtue of being recognized by antibodies, might function as mimics of antigens that would break tolerance instead of maintaining it—the so-called Ab2, used as antigen surrogates [32]. Thus a new context of molecular mimicry was born—one highlighted by the functionality of idiotypic antibodies in the context of the idiotype network theory [33–39].

Smaller fragments (peptides) of anti-idiotypes proved to translate successfully to vaccines too [40]. Peptides as mimics of antigens were clearly defined with the advent of phage screening technology [41, 42] growing in its application in biomedical sciences [43]. Peptide mimics are well defined as B and T cell epitopes [44]. Now there is an unprecedented opportunity to unravel the intricacies of the human immune response to immunization. Yet, fundamentally, vaccine strategies across susceptible disease depend on the identification of immunogenic antigens that can serve as the best targets [45–47].

Tumor antigens present a special challenge. Except for small details defined by mutations or altered post-translational modifications, generally they are self-antigens and this poses a barrier to effective vaccination. Tolerance is different from non-specific immunosuppression, and immunodeficiency. Like immune response, tolerance is specific existing both for T-cell and B cells and, like immunological memory tolerance is lasting longer at the T cell level than at the B cell level. Maintenance of immunological tolerance requires persistence of antigen. Tolerance can be broken naturally or artificially [48, 49]. Mimicry might impact on an already existing autoimmune process rather than precipitate novel disease by breaking of tolerance from the beginning [50]. While molecular mimicry is proposed as a basis for potential pathogenesis of some human disease, there are examples also of its exploitation in vaccine development.

3. Polyclonal activation

Now it is acknowledged that the natural antibody repertoire is created in the absence of exogenous antigens and/or germinal center maturation [51, 52]. It is also acknowledged that these preexisting antibodies can be affected by the presence of exogenous antigen since they recognize in a polyspecific manner evolutionarily fixed epitopes present in foreign antigens as well as on self-antigens [53]. Because of their constitutive expression, responses by natural antibodies are generally excluded from vaccine strategies. Among approaches that can modulate the natural antibody repertoire are immunizations affecting idiotypic interactions. When possible, an "idiotypic vaccination" could be a little explored way to activate the B and T cell cascades involving the natural responses against antigens.

Once acclaimed, idiotypy—the theory that the B lymphocyte repertoire forms a highly connected network of mutually recognizing and stimulating clones [54, 55]—unfortunately predated the discovery of many more levels of immune system complexity. The daunting task of attuning to the new knowledge prevented this theory from maintaining a support that would match its intellectual attractiveness. The first significant update, which almost rehabilitated it, stated that only the compartment of the B cell repertoire characterized by germline variable regions and the prerequisite physiological poly/autoreactivity forms this network [56]. Almost, because many immune system phenomena like a self-assertive rather than ignorant tolerance or the immune memory ultimately do not need to be explained by emergent properties of the immune network. Now it is accepted that specific cell populations and genetic programs rather than the dynamics of a network of functionally equivalent agents (clones) are responsible for almost all of the observed immune phenomena. In fact, recent development in our understanding of swarms of simple agents uncovers the limits of such systems where complexity of the behavior of the agents and the size of the system have Goldilocks conditions for optimal behavior [57]. No wonder, evolution has used the "swarm" solution rarely and ultimately replaced it (complemented it) in most cases by centralized systems and specialized components at a higher level of organization.

Another reason the intellectually attractive "second generation network" hypothesis also fails is may be the fact that the compartment producing natural antibodies is defined in many ways and even 25 years later is still rather a fuzzy set [53]. While the natural antibodies in a strict sense are produced by a particular subset of B1 cell derived plasma cells in the bone marrow without external stimulus there are B1 cells (e.g. B1b) and marginal zone cells that produce antibodies with many "natural" characteristics like polyspecificity in response to stimulation [58]. Thus, focusing on the naturally autoreactive compartment of the repertoire did not answer all questions but also added another dimension of uncertainty.

Natural antibodies are known to bind to a variety of antigens that are both self and exogenous and thereby providing one of the first lines of defense against both bacterial and viral pathogens [53, 59]. Antibodies reactive to self-antigens play a key role in both healthy individuals and patients with autoimmune disorders [60–62]. Hence, such antibodies are intrinsically multifaceted in their regulatory roles in immune responses and tolerance. While the immune response activated against self can be detrimental when triggered in an autoimmune genetic background, tuning immune activity with natural antibodies is a potential therapeutic strategy. One conceptual approach in this tuning is using naturally occurring anti-idiotype (anti-Id) antibodies to stimulate multifaceted natural antibodies.

4. Anti-idiotypic antibodies as mimics

Anti-idiotypic based vaccines have a long history of generating immune responses in experimental animals and in humans [27, 28, 63–65]. One of the first demonstrations for the basis of molecular mimicry observed between proteins and anti-idiotypes for proteins was dissected in the TEPC-15 idiotype system [66]. Vasta et al. [66] illustrated that mimicry could be at the sequence level. They suggested that the minimal stretch of homology (8–10 amino acid residues) was responsible for the cross-reactive nature of the TEPC-15 idiotype and the acute-phase protein C-reactive protein (CRP) from the horseshoe crab *Limulus polyphemus* (limulin). Of no less importance, it was shown that T helper cells could recognize a shared determinant that is present on idiotypically different myeloma proteins [67]. These findings collectively showed that T helper cells, induced by priming with antigen, can recognize shared idiotypic determinates, suggesting that peptides derived from anti-idiotypes can be processed as immunogens [40, 68].

The early studies of anti-idiotypes made clear the idea that functional mimicry of ligands of biological receptors is a matter of just binding to an antibody-binding site. This functional or antigenic mimicry ushered in concepts and a technology. It was evident that structural and immunological rules governing molecular mimicry require definition for its successful exploitation whether anti-idiotypes, small fragments derived from them or peptide mimetics [69, 70]. It was suggested that ligand-based pharmacophore design principles could be applied to designing peptides that can mimic ligands reactive with antibodies [69, 71]. Often times it was stated that there were no observable structural correlations to explain the mimicry [72]. Yet it seemed that antibodies could mimic antigens at the molecular level whereby the antigen and anti-idiotype could bind essentially the same combining-site residues of the Ab1 antibody [73].

Historically, clinical trials with anti-idiotypes in the cancer space have proved to be of mixed success [74, 75] but, clearly showing that humoral and cellular immune reactivity against a tumor can be enhanced upon active anti-id vaccination [76]. Other studies with anti-ids in humans have included those associated with tumor associated carbohydrate antigens (TACAs), [77–80]. An anti-Id vaccine, Racotumomab, raised against the murine anti-ganglioside N-glycolyl (NGc) GM3 (NGcGM3) has shown efficacy [81] in several phase I trials in melanoma, breast and lung cancers [82, 83]. These examples are representative for other anti-Id vaccine trials. In sum they indicate the induction of B and T-cell immune responses against a tumor.

5. Mimetic peptides in immuno-oncology

From a technology perspective the concept of developing and screening combinatorial or random peptide phage display became an effective means of identifying peptides that can bind target molecules and regulate their function [41, 42]. Phage-displayed peptide libraries have proved effective for (i) mapping of B and T cells epitopes, (ii) defining bioactive peptides that bind to receptors, (iii) selection of cell/organ specific binding peptides, and (iv) identification and development of peptide-mediated drug delivery systems to mention a few applications [43]. Among concepts emphasized by phage screening technology was that of the mimotope. The term mimotope, coined by Mario Geysen in 1986 [84] described a peptide mimicking a discontinuous antigenic determinant on foot and mouth virus. Phage screening technology has evolved, giving us unparalleled access to tight binding peptides to significantly accelerate identification of new leads for drug discovery [85].

The ability to produce combinatorial peptide libraries with a highly diverse pool of randomized ligands has transformed phage display into a straightforward, versatile and high throughput screening methodology for the identification of potential vaccine candidates against different diseases that include cancer [86–88]. While most studies with mimotopes identified by phage screening are still in preclinical studies, immunization results do provide insight for future development of novel mimotope-based tumor vaccines [89–92]. Starting from phage screening, we have developed carbohydrate-mimetic peptide (CMP) vaccines that target carbohydrate antigens [70, 71]. We brought CMPs from preclinical assessments of mimicking peptides of TACA [93–95] to clinical studies [17, 18] where one peptide can induce polyclonal responses to two or more antigens, which do or do not share epitopes.

Clinically we have shown that CMPs can achieve this multi-epitope targeting. The peptide P10s is a CMP designed to mimic both LeY and GD2 antigens using anti-LeY (BR55-2) and anti-GD2 (ME36.1) antibodies as templates [95]. Therefore, vaccination with P10s may lead to targeting various molecular entities associated with glycoproteins and with glycolipids, reducing the possibility of immune editing and escape. Moreover, the P10s vaccine has the potential to activate cellular responses [96]. We completed a phase I clinical trial of the P10s vaccine in breast cancer patients and showed its feasibility, safety and immune efficacy. The data indicates induction of anti-peptide and anti-glycan antibodies [17, 18]. Antibodies of immunized subjects mediated cytotoxicity on human breast cancer cell lines through currently unknown mechanisms independent of complement-mediated cell cytotoxicity, but had no effect on normal breast cell line MCF-10A [17, 18]. Serum antibodies parallel the effect of anti-LeY and anti-GD2 monoclonal antibodies. After more than 6 years of follow up, 4 out of 6 vaccinated subjects are still alive with 3 of them in remission. Our clinical data suggest that vaccination of breast cancer patient's results in tumor regression and survival benefit.

6. Linking signaling with polyclonal response

The complexity of glycans found on the cell surface argues for their informational role involved in regulating multiple cellular processes essential for tumor development or its metastases. Since TACAs are expressed on glycoproteins and glycolipids that regulate multiple cellular pathways, TACAs are by definition pan-targets. Many glycoproteins and glycolipids are associated with signaling cascades through Focal Adhesion Kinase (FAK) with its activation hypothesized to play an important role in the pathogenesis of human cancers [97, 98]. FAK is a non-receptor tyrosine kinase that plays an important role in signal transduction pathways that are initiated at sites of integrin-mediated cell adhesion and by growth factor receptors [99]. FAK is also linked to oncogenes at both a biochemical and functional level. Moreover, overexpression and/or increased activity of FAK are common in a wide variety of human cancers, implicating a role for FAK in carcinogenesis. It is therefore a key regulator of survival, proliferation, migration and invasion: signaling cascades and processes that are all involved in the development and progression of cancer. FAK localized at focal contact sites and communicates with TACA-expressing molecules. Coordinated and localized stimulation of these cascades influences focal contact turnover and actin cytoskeleton dynamic addition to expression of motility- and invasion-associated proteins such as matrix metalloproteinases. FAK-dependent regulation of chemokine's and cytokines in cancer cells can drive elevated levels of regulatory T cells into the tumor environment resulting in suppression of the anti-tumor CD8+ T-cell response [100].

FAK is associated with several mechanisms to regulate cell migration and invasion through its phosphorylation. These include interactions with Src, P13K, Grb7, N-WASP and EndoII. Interaction with integrin also mediates FAK association with extracellular matrix, triggering the binding of adaptor molecules leading to the modulation of small GTPases, Ack, ERK2/MAP and JNK/SAP kinase cascades. The convergence of signaling by FAK plays an important role in tumor-cell survival and in drug resistance, as these pathways overlap. Given the important role of FAK in a large number of processes involved in tumorigenesis, metastasis, and survival signaling, Akt/FAK pathways are now regarded as a potential target to overcome drug resistance.

A variety of results suggest that GD2 and LeY play a role in the migration and survival of cancer cells, since (i) anti-GD2 antibodies [101] and natural anti-TACA antibodies [102] can mediate anoikis; (ii) apoptosis signals are transduced via reduction in the phosphorylation levels of FAK, the activation of a MAPK family members, p38 and c-Jun terminal kinase (JNK), upon binding of such antibodies [101, 103]; (iii) P10s reacts with anti-GD2 and anti-LeY monoclonal antibodies; (iv) anti-P10s antibodies block cell migration and (v) anti-P10s antibodies from P10s immunized subjects are cytotoxic to human breast cancer cell lines.

7. Synergism of chemo- and immunotherapy

Combining agents with distinct or perhaps overlapping mechanisms of action can potentially result in synergistic anticancer effects. Numerous preclinical studies have established the synergistic relationships between modulation of Tregs and differential expression of immune effector ligands on tumor cells [104, 105]. Consequently, combinatorial anticancer therapy is now a well-established paradigm due to a number of clinical trials demonstrating therapeutic success. However, the mechanisms associated with successful application are not well understood [106]. Standard cancer chemotherapy can promote tumor immunity in two major ways: (i) inducing immunogenic cell death as part of its intended therapeutic effect leading to epitope spreading [107, 108]; and (ii) disrupting strategies that tumors use to evade the immune response [109, 110]. In particular, epitope spreading ensures a polyclonal, polyfunctional immune response that promises to keep the tumor in check indefinitely [111]. Cancer patients can display tumor-reactive antibodies at baseline, which can increase in both breadth and quantity after immunotherapy [112]. IgG antibodies, produced by B cells, are indicative of CD4 helper T cells of linked specificity. Activation of tumor-specific CD8 T cells result from the same processes that generate activated CD4 T cells.

Checkpoint inhibitors have changed the face of immunotherapy with objective responses observed in some patients based on combinatorial regimes involving CTLA4 agent ipilimumab and the PD-1-specific checkpoint inhibitor nivolumab [113]. Nevertheless, a sizeable fraction of patients do not respond to checkpoint inhibitor combination. This could be for several reasons that include but are not limited to not having the correct T cell precursors to target the tumor associated antigens, dysfunctional T cell receptors and down regulation of MHC complexes [114, 115]. Interestingly, FAK inhibition has been noted to increase the activity of checkpoint inhibitors [116]. This work suggests that FAK inhibition increases immune surveillance and renders tumors responsive to immunotherapy.

In our own work when combining chemotherapy with CMPs we primarily focused on immune effector synergistic relationships. A particular synergistic action requires apoptotic tumor cell death, and does not occur as a consequence of perturbations in immunological regulatory circuits. The resistance of many types of cancer to conventional chemotherapies is problematic and a major factor undermining successful cancer treatment. Again FAK plays a role with its silencing augments docetaxel-mediated apoptosis of cancer cells [117]. We have shown that immunization with P10s can overcome resistance to taxanes and coupled with other studies indicating that targeting GD2 antigen is associated with FAK silencing we have come to another important therapeutic option of inducing multiple responses that go through the FAK gatekeeper to improve upon immunotherapy strategies.

8. Conclusion

Harnessing the body's own immune system to kill cancer cells has shown promise for a growing number of cancers, revolutionizing the clinical management of multiple tumors. The success of checkpoint antagonists heralds the dawn of a new age in cancer therapy, in which immunotherapy is becoming a key strategy for clinical management. Checkpoint inhibitors have taught us that they can unleash natural responses to tumor cells. The goal of cancer vaccines should be rethought in terms of boosting those natural responses. Combination therapies that integrate distinct therapeutic modalities that include vaccines, small molecules, radiotherapy and checkpoint inhibitors are under investigation. Yet understanding the cellular and molecular underpins are essential for effective translation to the clinic. Polyclonal activation of the immune system should lend to epitope spreading phenomena, which will further effectiveness of cancer therapy. Yet this concept had been for the most part limited to the idea of presenting multiple epitopes of a particular target associated with T cell activation. This viewpoint needs to be reassessed to include the idea of extending to humoral responses since antibodies have proved to be essential to the cancer treating armament.

Conflict of interest

The authors declare that this research was conducted in the absence of any commercial or financial relationships that could be construed as a potential conflict of interest. TKE and AP are named as inventors on an institutional patent application filled by UAMS that is related to the CMP vaccine briefly described in this manuscript. Therefore, TKE and AP and UAMS have a potential financial interest in the vaccine briefly described. No financial or other support of any kind has resulted from this patent application. These financial interests have been reviewed by approved supervision in accordance with the UAMS conflict of interest policies.

Author details

Anastas Pashov[1] and Thomas Kieber-Emmons[2]*

1 Stephan Angelov Institute of Microbiology, Bulgarian Academy of Sciences, Sofia, Bulgaria

2 Winthrop P. Rockefeller Cancer Institute, Department of Pathology, University of Arkansas for Medical Sciences, Little Rock, AR, USA

*Address all correspondence to: tke@uams.edu

IntechOpen

© 2019 The Author(s). Licensee IntechOpen. This chapter is distributed under the terms of the Creative Commons Attribution License (http://creativecommons.org/licenses/by/3.0), which permits unrestricted use, distribution, and reproduction in any medium, provided the original work is properly cited. CC BY

References

[1] Pardoll D. Cancer and the immune system: Basic concepts and targets for intervention. Seminars in Oncology. 2015;**42**(4):523-538. DOI: 10.1053/j.seminoncol.2015.05.003. Epub 2015 Jun 3

[2] Sabado RL, Bhardwaj N. Directing dendritic cell immunotherapy towards successful cancer treatment. Immunotherapy. 2010;**2**(1):37-56. DOI: 10.2217/imt.09.43

[3] Gardner A, Ruffell B. Dendritic cells and cancer immunity. Trends in Immunology. 2016;**37**(12):855-865. DOI: 10.1016/j.it.2016.09.006. Epub 2016 Oct 25

[4] Mackiewicz J et al. Re-induction using whole cell melanoma vaccine genetically modified to melanoma stem cells-like beyond recurrence extends long term survival of high risk resected patients—Updated results. Journal for ImmunoTherapy of Cancer. 2018;**6**(1):134. DOI: 10.1186/s40425-018-0456-1

[5] Kwiatkowska-Borowczyk E et al. Whole cell melanoma vaccine genetically modified to stem cells like phenotype generates specific immune responses to ALDH1A1 and long-term survival in advanced melanoma patients. Oncoimmunology. 2018;**7**(11):e1509821. DOI: 10.1080/2162402X.2018.1509821. eCollection 2018

[6] Monzavi-Karbassi B, Pashov A, Kieber-Emmons T. Tumor-associated glycans and immune surveillance. Vaccines (Basel). 2013;**1**(2):174-203. DOI: 10.3390/vaccines1020174

[7] Sadraei SI, Reynolds MR, Trant JF. The synthesis and biological characterization of acetal-free mimics of the tumor-associated carbohydrate antigens. Advances in Carbohydrate Chemistry and Biochemistry. 2017;**74**:137-237. DOI: 10.1016/bs.accb.2017.10.003. Epub 2017 Nov 20

[8] Liu CC, Ye XS. Carbohydrate-based cancer vaccines: Target cancer with sugar bullets. Glycoconjugate Journal. 2012;**29**(5-6):259-271. DOI: 10.1007/s10719-012-9399-9. Epub 2012 Jun 6

[9] Wei MM, Wang YS, Ye XS. Carbohydrate-based vaccines for oncotherapy. Medicinal Research Reviews. 2018;**38**(3):1003-1026. DOI: 10.1002/med.21493. Epub 2018 Mar 7

[10] Hahn AW et al. The future of immune checkpoint cancer therapy after PD-1 and CTLA-4. Immunotherapy. 2017;**9**(8):681-692. DOI: 10.2217/imt-2017-0024

[11] Emerson DA, Redmond WL. Overcoming tumor-induced immune suppression: From relieving inhibition to providing costimulation with T cell agonists. BioDrugs. 2018;**32**(3):221-231. DOI: 10.1007/s40259-018-0277-2

[12] Du X et al. A reappraisal of CTLA-4 checkpoint blockade in cancer immunotherapy. Cell Research. 2018;**28**(4):416-432. DOI: 10.1038/s41422-018-0011-0. Epub 2018 Feb 22

[13] Pashov A et al. Thinking cancer. Monoclonal Antibodies in Immunodiagnosis and Immunotherapy. 2018;**37**(3):117-125. DOI: 10.1089/mab.2018.0014

[14] Gross S et al. Targeting cancer with kinase inhibitors. The Journal of Clinical Investigation. 2015;**125**(5):1780-1789. DOI: 10.1172/JCI76094. Epub 2015 May 1

[15] Rodon J et al. Development of PI3K inhibitors: Lessons learned from early clinical trials. Nature Reviews. Clinical Oncology. 2013;**10**(3):143-153. DOI: 10.1038/nrclinonc.2013.10. Epub 2013 Feb 12

[16] Tsao CY et al. Anti-proliferative and pro-apoptotic activity of GD2 ganglioside-specific monoclonal antibody 3F8 in human melanoma cells. Oncoimmunology. 2015;**4**(8):e1023975. DOI: 10.1080/2162402X.2015.1023975. eCollection 2015 Aug

[17] Hutchins LF et al. Targeting tumor-associated carbohydrate antigens: A phase I study of a carbohydrate mimetic-peptide vaccine in stage IV breast cancer subjects. Oncotarget. 2017;**8**(58): 99161-99178. DOI: 10.18632/oncotarget.21959. eCollection 2017 Nov 17

[18] Makhoul I et al. Moving a carbohydrate mimetic peptide into the clinic. Human Vaccines & Immunotherapeutics. 2015;**11**(1):37-44. DOI: 10.4161/hv.34300. Epub 2014 Nov 1

[19] Clay TM et al. Polyclonal immune responses to antigens associated with cancer signaling pathways and new strategies to enhance cancer vaccines. Immunologic Research. 2011;**49**(1-3):235-247. DOI: 10.1007/s12026-010-8186-6

[20] Cohn M. Ten experiments that would make a difference in understanding immune mechanisms. Cellular and Molecular Life Sciences. 2012;**69**(3):405-412. DOI: 10.1007/s00018-011-0869-1. Epub 2011 Nov 1

[21] Davis MM, Tato CM, Furman D. Systems immunology: Just getting started. Nature Immunology. 2017;**18**(7):725-732. DOI: 10.1038/ni.3768

[22] Villani AC, Sarkizova S, Hacohen N. Systems immunology: Learning the rules of the immune system. Annual Review of Immunology. 2018;**36**:813-842. DOI: 10.1146/annurev-immunol-042617-053035

[23] Wooden SL, Koff WC. The human vaccines project: Towards a comprehensive understanding of the human immune response to immunization. Human Vaccines & Immunotherapeutics. 2018;**14**(9):2214-2216. DOI: 10.1080/21645515.2018.1476813. Epub 2018 Jun 28

[24] Coutinho A. The self-nonself discrimination and the nature and acquisition of the antibody repertoire. Annales d'immunologie. 1980;**131D**(3):235-253

[25] Isenberg D, Shoenfeld Y. Autoantibodies, idiotypes, anti-idiotypes and autoimmunity. Acta Haematologica. 1986;**76**(2-3):95-100

[26] Vertosick FT, Kelly RH. The immune system as a neural network: A multi-epitope approach. Journal of Theoretical Biology. 1991;**150**(2):225-237

[27] Lopez-Requena A, Burrone OR, Cesco-Gaspere M. Idiotypes as immunogens: Facing the challenge of inducing strong therapeutic immune responses against the variable region of immunoglobulins. Frontiers in Oncology. 2012;**2**:159. DOI: 10.3389/fonc.2012.00159. eCollection 2012

[28] Kieber-Emmons T et al. The promise of the anti-idiotype concept. Frontiers in Oncology. 2012;**2**(196):1-12. DOI: 10.3389/fonc.2012.00196. eCollection 02012

[29] Adib M et al. IgG autoantibody activity in normal mouse serum is controlled by IgM. Journal of Immunology. 1990;**145**(11):3807-3813

[30] Hurez V et al. Pooled normal human polyspecific IgM contains neutralizing anti-idiotypes to IgG autoantibodies of autoimmune patients and protects from experimental autoimmune disease. Blood. 1997;**90**(10):4004-4013

[31] Quaglia S et al. A functional idiotype/anti-idiotype network is

active in genetically gluten-intolerant individuals negative for both celiac disease–related intestinal damage and serum autoantibodies. The Journal of Immunology. 2019;**202**(4):1079-1087

[32] Kohler H. The servant idiotype network. Scandinavian Journal of Immunology. 1991;**33**(5):495-497 discussion 498

[33] Augustin AA, Sim GK, Bona CA. Internal images of antigens within the immune network. Survey of Immunologic Research. 1983;**2**(1):78-87

[34] Bona CA. Internal image concept revisited. Proceedings of the Society for Experimental Biology and Medicine. 1996;**213**(1):32-42

[35] Bona CA et al. Epibody: The image of the network created by a single antibody. Immunological Reviews. 1986;**90**:115-127

[36] Geha RS. Idiotypic-antiidiotypic interactions in humans. Journal of Biological Response Modifiers. 1984;**3**(6):573-579

[37] Kennedy RC, Melnick JL, Dreesman GR. Anti-idiotypes and immunity. Scientific American. 1986;**255**(1):48-56

[38] Cheng HL et al. Structural basis of stimulatory anti-idiotypic antibodies. Molecular Immunology. 1988;**25**(1):33-40

[39] Kohler H et al. Idiotypic networks and nature of molecular mimicry: An overview. Methods in Enzymology. 1989;**178**:3-35

[40] Westerink MA et al. Peptide mimicry of the meningococcal group C capsular polysaccharide. Proceedings of the National Academy of Sciences of the United States of America. 1995;**92**(9):4021-4025

[41] Smith G. Filamentous fusion phage: Novel expression vectors that display cloned antigens on the virion surface. Science. 1985;**228**(4705):1315-1317

[42] Smith GP. Surface presentation of protein epitopes using bacteriophage expression systems. Current Opinion in Biotechnology. 1991;**2**(5):668-673

[43] Wu CH et al. Advancement and applications of peptide phage display technology in biomedical science. Journal of Biomedical Science. 2016;**23**(8):1-14. DOI: 10.1186/s12929-016-0223-x

[44] Pinilla C, et al. Identification of B cell and T cell epitopes using synthetic peptide combinatorial libraries. Current Protocols in Immunology. 2012;Chapter(9): p. Unit9.5. DOI: 10.1002/0471142735.im0905s99

[45] Finn OJ. Human tumor antigens yesterday, today, and tomorrow. Cancer Immunology Research. 2017;**5**(5):347-354. DOI: 10.1158/2326-6066.CIR-17-0112

[46] Wang RF, Wang HY. Immune targets and neoantigens for cancer immunotherapy and precision medicine. Cell Research. 2017;**27**(1):11-37. DOI: 10.1038/cr.2016.155. Epub 2016 Dec 27

[47] Siniard RC, Harada S. Immunogenomics: Using genomics to personalize cancer immunotherapy. Virchows Archiv. 2017;**417**:209-219

[48] Prinz JC. Disease mimicry—A pathogenetic concept for T cell-mediated autoimmune disorders triggered by molecular mimicry? Autoimmunity Reviews. 2004;**3**(1):10-15. DOI: 10.1016/S1568-9972(03)00059-4

[49] Oldstone MB. Molecular mimicry: Its evolution from concept to mechanism as a cause of

autoimmune diseases. Monoclonal Antibodies in Immunodiagnosis and Immunotherapy. 2014;**33**(3):158-165. DOI: 10.1089/mab.2013.0090. Epub 2014 Apr 2

[50] Rojas M et al. Molecular mimicry and autoimmunity. Journal of Autoimmunity. 2018;**95**:100-123. DOI: 10.1016/j.jaut.2018.10.012. Epub 2018 Oct 26

[51] Hooijkaas H et al. Isotypes and specificities of immunoglobulins produced by germ-free mice fed chemically defined ultrafiltered "antigen-free" diet. European Journal of Immunology. 1984;**14**(12):1127-1130

[52] Baumgarth N. How specific is too specific? B-cell responses to viral infections reveal the importance of breadth over depth. Immunological Reviews. 2013;**255**(1):82-94

[53] Holodick NE, Rodríguez-Zhurbenko N, Hernández AM. Defining natural antibodies. Frontiers in Immunology. 2017;**8**:872

[54] Jerne NK. Towards a network theory of the immune system. Annales d'Immunologie (Paris). 1974;**125C**(1-2):373-389

[55] Jerne NK. The immune system: A web of V-domains. Harvey Lectures. 1974;**70**:93-110

[56] Varela F, Coutinho A. Second generation immune networks. Immunology Today. 1991;**12**:159-166

[57] Manrique PD et al. Getting closer to the goal by being less capable. Science Advances. 2019;**5**(2):eaau5902

[58] Savage HP, Baumgarth N. Characteristics of natural antibody-secreting cells. Annals of the New York Academy of Sciences. 2015;**1362**:132-142

[59] Vale AM et al. The global self-reactivity profile of the natural antibody repertoire is largely independent of germline DH sequence. Frontiers in Immunology. 2016;**7**:296. DOI: 10.3389/fimmu.2016.00296. eCollection 2016

[60] Lundkvist I et al. Evidence for a functional idiotypic network among natural antibodies in normal mice. Proceedings of the National Academy of Sciences of the United States of America. 1989;**86**:5074-5078

[61] Baumgarth N et al. The role of B-1 and B-2 cells in immune protection from influenza virus infection. Current Topics in Microbiology and Immunology. 2000;**252**:163-169

[62] Nguyen TT, Elsner RA, Baumgarth N. Natural IgM prevents autoimmunity by enforcing B cell central tolerance induction. Journal of Immunology. 2015;**194**(4):1489-1502

[63] Kohler H et al. Revised immune network concepts. Clinical Immunology and Immunopathology. 1989;**52**(1):104-116

[64] Ruffini PA et al. Idiotypic vaccination for B-cell malignancies as a model for therapeutic cancer vaccines: From prototype protein to second generation vaccines. Haematologica. 2002;**87**(9):989-1001

[65] de Cerio AL et al. Anti-idiotype antibodies in cancer treatment. Oncogene. 2007;**26**(25):3594-3602

[66] Vasta GR, Marchalonis JJ, Kohler H. Invertebrate recognition protein cross-reacts with an immunoglobulin idiotype. The Journal of Experimental Medicine. 1984;**159**(4):1270-1276

[67] Gleason K, Kohler H. Regulatory idiotypes. T helper cells recognize a shared VH idiotope on phosphorylcholine-specific antibodies.

The Journal of Experimental Medicine. 1982;**156**(2):539-549

[68] Raychaudhuri S et al. Tumor idiotype vaccines. VII. Analysis and correlation of structural, idiotypic, and biologic properties of protective and nonprotective Ab2. Journal of Immunology. 1990;**145**(2):760-767

[69] Kieber-Emmons T et al. Structural considerations in idiotype vaccine design. Monographs in Allergy. 1987;**22**:126-133

[70] Cunto-Amesty G et al. Exploiting molecular mimicry: Defining rules of the game. International Reviews of Immunology. 2001;**20**(2):157-180

[71] Luo P et al. A molecular basis for functional peptide mimicry of a carbohydrate antigen. The Journal of Biological Chemistry. 2000;**275**(21):16146-16154

[72] Bentley GA et al. Three-dimensional structure of an idiotope-anti-idiotope complex. Nature. 1990;**348**(6298):254-257

[73] Fields BA et al. Molecular basis of antigen mimicry by an anti-idiotope. Nature. 1995;**374**(6524):739-742

[74] Herlyn D et al. Anti-idiotype cancer vaccines: Past and future. Cancer Immunology, Immunotherapy. 1996;**43**(2):65-76

[75] Foon KA et al. Immune response to the carcinoembryonic antigen in patients treated with an anti-idiotype antibody vaccine. The Journal of Clinical Investigation. 1995;**96**(1):334-342

[76] Herlyn D et al. Anti-idiotype immunization of cancer patients: Modulation of the immune response. Proceedings of the National Academy of Sciences of the United States of America. 1987;**84**(22):8055-8059

[77] McCaffery M et al. Immunization of melanoma patients with BEC2 anti-idiotypic monoclonal antibody that mimics GD3 ganglioside: Enhanced immunogenicity when combined with adjuvant. Clinical Cancer Research. 1996;**2**(4):679-686

[78] Yao TJ et al. Immunization of melanoma patients with BEC2-keyhole limpet hemocyanin plus BCG intradermally followed by intravenous booster immunizations with BEC2 to induce anti-GD3 ganglioside antibodies. Clinical Cancer Research. 1999;**5**(1):77-81

[79] Grant SC et al. Long survival of patients with small cell lung cancer after adjuvant treatment with the anti-idiotypic antibody BEC2 plus Bacillus Calmette-Guerin. Clinical Cancer Research. 1999;**5**(6):1319-1323

[80] Foon KA et al. Clinical and immune responses in advanced melanoma patients immunized with an anti-idiotype antibody mimicking disialoganglioside GD2. Journal of Clinical Oncology. 2000;**18**(2):376-384. DOI: 10.1200/JCO.2000.18.2.376

[81] Perez A et al. A monoclonal antibody against NeuGc-containing gangliosides contains a regulatory idiotope involved in the interaction with B and T cells. Molecular Immunology. 2002;**39**(1-2):103-112

[82] Diaz A et al. Immune responses in breast cancer patients immunized with an anti-idiotype antibody mimicking NeuGc-containing gangliosides. Clinical Immunology. 2003;**107**(2):80-89

[83] Neninger E et al. Active immunotherapy with 1E10 anti-idiotype vaccine in patients with small cell lung cancer: Report of a phase I trial. Cancer Biology & Therapy. 2007;**6**(2):145-150

[84] Geysen HM, Rodda SJ, Mason TJ. A priori delineation of a peptide which mimics a discontinuous antigenic determinant. Molecular Immunology. 1986;**23**(7):709-715

[85] Obexer R, Walport LJ, Suga H. Exploring sequence space: Harnessing chemical and biological diversity towards new peptide leads. Current Opinion in Chemical Biology. 2017;**38**:52-61. DOI: 10.1016/j.cbpa.2017.02.020. Epub 2017 Mar 17

[86] Aghebati-Maleki L et al. Phage display as a promising approach for vaccine development. Journal of Biomedical Science. 2016;**23**(1):66

[87] Goulart LR, Santos Pde S. Strategies for vaccine design using phage display-derived peptides. Methods in Molecular Biology. 2016;**1404**:423-435. DOI: 10.1007/978-1-4939-3389-1_28

[88] Huang J, He B, Zhou P. Mimotope-based prediction of B-cell epitopes. Methods in Molecular Biology. 2014;**1184**:237-243. DOI: 10.1007/978-1-4939-1115-8_13

[89] Orlandi R et al. Antigenic and immunogenic mimicry of the HER2/neu oncoprotein by phage-displayed peptides. European Journal of Immunology. 1994;**24**(11):2868-2873

[90] Zhao L, Liu Z, Fan D. Overview of mimotopes and related strategies in tumor vaccine development. Expert Review of Vaccines. 2008;**7**(10):1547-1555. DOI: 10.1586/14760584.7.10.1547

[91] Ashok BT et al. Peptide mimotopes of oncoproteins as therapeutic agents in breast cancer. International Journal of Molecular Medicine. 2003;**11**(4):465-471

[92] Sherev T, Wiesmuller KH, Walden P. Mimotopes of tumor-associated T-cell epitopes for cancer vaccines determined with combinatorial peptide libraries. Molecular Biotechnology. 2003;**25**(1):53-61

[93] Agadjanyan M et al. Peptide mimicry of carbohydrate epitopes on human immunodeficiency virus. Nature Biotechnology. 1997;**15**(6):547-551. DOI: 10.1038/nbt0697-547

[94] Kieber-Emmons T et al. Vaccination with carbohydrate peptide mimotopes promotes anti-tumor responses. Nature Biotechnology. 1999;**17**(7):660-665. DOI: 10.1038/10870

[95] Monzavi-Karbassi B et al. Preclinical studies of carbohydrate mimetic peptide vaccines for breast cancer and melanoma. Vaccine. 2007;**25**(16):3022-3031. DOI: 10.1016/j.vaccine.2007.01.072. Epub 2007 Jan 26

[96] Wondimu A et al. Peptides mimicking GD2 ganglioside elicit cellular, humoral and tumor-protective immune responses in mice. Cancer Immunology, Immunotherapy. 2008;**57**(7):1079-1089

[97] Zhao X, Guan JL. Focal adhesion kinase and its signaling pathways in cell migration and angiogenesis. Advanced Drug Delivery Reviews. 2011;**63**(8):610-615. DOI: 10.1016/j.addr.2010.11.001. Epub 2010 Nov 29

[98] Tai YL, Chen LC, Shen TL. Emerging roles of focal adhesion kinase in cancer. BioMed Research International. 2015;**2015**:690690. DOI: 10.1155/2015/690690. Epub 2015 Mar 31

[99] Guan JL. Integrin signaling through FAK in the regulation of mammary stem cells and breast cancer. IUBMB Life. 2010;**62**(4):268-276. DOI: 10.1002/iub.303

[100] Serrels A et al. Nuclear FAK controls chemokine transcription, Tregs, and evasion of anti-tumor immunity. Cell. 2015;**163**(1):160-173. DOI: 10.1016/j.cell.2015.09.001

[101] Aixinjueluo W et al. Mechanisms for the apoptosis of small cell lung cancer cells induced by anti-GD2 monoclonal antibodies: Roles of anoikis. The Journal of Biological Chemistry. 2005;**280**(33):29828-29836. Epub 2005 May 26

[102] Vollmers HP, Brandlein S. Natural antibodies and cancer. New Biotechnology. 2009;**25**(5):294-298. Epub 2009 Apr 11

[103] Yoshida S et al. An anti-GD2 monoclonal antibody enhances apoptotic effects of anti-cancer drugs against small cell lung cancer cells via JNK (c-Jun terminal kinase) activation. Japanese Journal of Cancer Research. 2002;**93**(7):816-824

[104] Ribas A. Anti-CTLA4 antibody clinical trials in melanoma. Update on Cancer Therapeutics. 2007;**2**(3):133-139

[105] Asano T et al. PD-1 modulates regulatory T-cell homeostasis during low-dose interleukin-2 therapy. Blood. 2017;**129**(15):2186-2197

[106] Emens LA, Middleton G. The interplay of immunotherapy and chemotherapy: Harnessing potential synergies. Cancer Immunology Research. 2015;**3**(5):436-443. DOI: 10.1158/2326-6066.CIR-15-0064

[107] Tesniere A et al. Molecular characteristics of immunogenic cancer cell death. Cell Death and Differentiation. 2008;**15**(1):3-12

[108] Pfirschke C et al. Immunogenic chemotherapy sensitizes tumors to checkpoint blockade therapy. Immunity. 2016;**44**(2):343-354

[109] Baitsch L et al. The three main stumbling blocks for anticancer T cells. Trends in Immunology. Jul 2012;**33**(7):364-372. DOI: 10.1016/j.it.2012.02.006

[110] Takeuchi Y, Nishikawa H. Roles of regulatory T cells in cancer immunity. International Immunology. 2016;**28**(8):401-409

[111] Heckler M, Dougan SK. Unmasking pancreatic cancer: Epitope spreading after single antigen chimeric antigen receptor T-cell therapy in a human phase I trial. Gastroenterology. 2018;**155**(1): 11-14. DOI: 10.1053/j.gastro.2018.06.023. Epub 2018 Jun 6

[112] Gnjatic S et al. Identifying baseline immune-related biomarkers to predict clinical outcome of immunotherapy. Journal for ImmunoTherapy of Cancer. 2017;**5**:44. DOI: 10.1186/s40425-017-0243-4. eCollection 2017

[113] Kroemer G, Galluzzi L. Combinatorial immunotherapy with checkpoint blockers solves the problem of metastatic melanoma—An exclamation sign with a question mark. Oncoimmunology. 2015;**4**(7):e1058037. DOI: 10.1080/2162402X.2015.1058037. eCollection 2015 Jul

[114] De Sousa Linhares A et al. Not all immune checkpoints are created equal. Frontiers in Immunology. 31 Aug 2018;**9**(1909):1-15. DOI: 10.3389/fimmu.2018.01909. eCollection 2018

[115] Park JA, Cheung N-KV. Limitations and opportunities for immune checkpoint inhibitors in pediatric malignancies. Cancer Treatment Reviews. 2017;**58**:22-33

[116] Jiang H et al. Targeting focal adhesion kinase renders pancreatic cancers responsive to checkpoint immunotherapy. Nature Medicine. 2016;**22**(8):851-860. DOI: 10.1038/nm.4123. Epub 2016 Jul 4

[117] Halder J et al. Focal adhesion kinase silencing augments docetaxel-mediated apoptosis in ovarian cancer cells. Clinical Cancer Research. 2005;**11**(24 Pt 1):8829-8836. DOI: 10.1158/1078-0432.CCR-05-1728

Chapter 4

Natural Killer (NK) Cell Alloreactivities against Leukemic Cells: Functions beyond Defense

Suwit Chaisri and Chanvit Leelayuwat

Abstract

Immunotherapy using adoptive transfer of natural killer (NK) cells has progressively been utilized in hematologic malignancies over the past decade. Presently, NK cell immunotherapy has been promising and feasible in acute leukemia, particularly in acute myeloblastic leukemia (AML). Alloreactive NK cells have been exploited under the killer immunoglobulin-like receptor (KIR)-ligand mismatches between donors and recipients in haploidentical hematopoietic stem cell transplantation (haplo-HSCT) after immunosuppressive chemotherapy. Of interest, alloreactive NK cells killed residual leukemic cells, dendritic cells (DCs) and T cells in acute leukemia patients and led to significantly improved clinical outcomes. Consequently, this chapter provides the *KIR* genetics and the mechanisms of alloreactive NK cells that are shown to be crucial in the successful therapy of acute leukemia (myeloid and lymphoid). Altogether, the donor selection algorithm of haplo-HSCT is discussed to emphasize the importance and give priority to increase the chances of therapy success. These will be useful for students and researchers who work in immunogenetics. Furthermore, the knowledge would be applicable to clinical research and medical sciences.

Keywords: NK cell alloreactivity, *KIR* polymorphisms, KIR-ligands mismatch, acute leukemia, haploidentical HSCT

1. Introduction

Natural killer (NK) cells play a critical role in innate immune responses against infected cells and transformed cells. In the past decades, the molecular mechanisms of NK cell killings have been extensively elucidated as well as employed in clinical applications [1, 2]. The effector functions of NK cells are being investigated in several pathological conditions, particularly in cancers [3, 4]. Many researches highlight on the role of NK cells in hematologic malignancies, particularly in acute leukemia. Acute leukemia is a type of cancer in which the bone marrow produces too many immature white blood cells and they cannot carry out normal functions. In addition, leukemic cells crowd out all blood cell productions in the bone marrow, affecting normal blood functions and leading to serious health problems. The treatment options for acute leukemia include chemotherapy, radiotherapy and bone marrow (hematopoietic stem cell) transplantation. Considering HLA matching between donors and patients for hematopoietic stem cell transplantation (HSCT),

IntechOpen

the patient's outcomes are related with a closely matched donor, however, not all patients are able to find a suitable donor. To overcome the limitations of donor availability, a partially matched or haploidentical HSCT (haplo-HSCT) has been established as an alternative expedient and being a mode of curative therapy for hematologic malignancies [5], particularly in acute leukemia patients [6]. In addition, a complication of allogeneic HSCT has improved with graft versus host disease (GvHD) prophylaxis to prevent the effects of donor T cells. Evidently, the role of NK cell alloreactivity can significantly improve clinical outcomes in acute leukemia patients [7]. Among NK cell receptors, killer immunoglobulin-like receptor (KIR) has increasingly been exploited in the aspect of immunotherapy for acute leukemia, which mismatches between KIR on donor NK cells and their cognate ligand HLA class I on receipts lead to alloreactivity of NK cells in haplo-HSCT setting. Alloreactive NK cells exert powerful activity in killing residual leukemic cells, leading to preventing disease relapse and improving survival [7, 8]. With these reasons, NK cell alloreactivities mediated by KIR-ligand mismatches has been increasingly utilized in aspect of immunotherapy for clinical applications. Therefore, this chapter provides *KIR* genetics and KIR-mediated NK cell alloreactivities that have been shown to be crucial in the successful therapy of acute leukemia (myeloid and lymphoid). Additionally, donor selection algorithm of haploidentical HSCT mismatch is discussed to emphasize its role in increasing success rate of these therapies.

2. Natural killer (NK) cells

NK cells are considered a part of lymphocytes that account for approximately 10% of blood lymphocytes. NK cells are characterized by expression of CD56 surface antigen and a lack of CD3 antigen. Based on the density of CD56 expression, human NK cells are phenotypically divided into two groups: $CD56^{bright}$ and $CD56^{dim}$. Of these NK cell populations, $CD56^{dim}$ NK cells represent up to 90% of NK cells in human peripheral blood mononuclear cells (PBMCs) and are considered the most cytotoxic subset, while CD 56^{bright} NK cells comprise approximately 10% of NK cells in PBMCs and are known as the cytokine-producing subset. NK cells play important role of the first line of defense to infected cells and transformed cells without prior sensitization [9, 10]. Several receptors present on NK cells are currently identified, however, they are classified into two groups depended on signal transductions derived from those receptors, namely activating and inhibitory receptors [11] (**Table 1**). Importantly, the dynamic equilibrium of signals obtained by these receptors is important to determine whether NK cells are activated to kill target cells [12, 13]. The missing self-hypothesis has been proposed to explain whether NK cells discriminate target cells form healthy "self" cells by their various receptors [14]. Normally, engagement of inhibitory receptors by self MHC class I molecule leads to transmission of an inhibitory signal to switch off the NK cell functions, while down-regulated MHC molecules on target cells by viral infection or malignant transformation is recognized and attacked by NK cells. Cytotoxicity and cytokine secretion of NK cells depended on the interaction between their receptors and their corresponding ligands. Activated NK cells usually exert cytotoxic activity through three main pathways. Firstly, the perforin/granzymes pathway, activated NK cells release these molecules to intracellular space. The perforin directly forms a transmembrane channel on the target cell, leading to increased permeability of the target cell membrane and causing osmotic lyses of target cells. In addition, granzymes enter the cytoplasm of target cells through transmembrane pores to promote target cells apoptosis [15]. Secondly, the Fas/FasL pathway, when Fas on NK cells binds to FasL on the target cells, Fas derivers a death signal to the target cell

Type of receptors	Ligands
Activating receptors	
CD94-NKG2C/E	HLA-E
NKG2D	MIC-A/-B, ULBP1–6
KIR-S	HLA-C
NKp30	B7H6, BAT3
NKp44	Proteoglycans
NKp46	Heparin
CD16	IgG
Inhibitory receptors	
KIR-L	HLA-A, -B, -C
LAIR-1	Collagen
LILRB1	HLA-A, -B, -C
NKR	LLT-1
KLRG1	Cadherins
SIGLEC3, 7,9	Sialic acid
CD94-NKG2A	HLA-E
Activating or inhibitory receptors	
KIR2DL4	HLA-G?

KIR-S: killer cell immunoglobulin-like receptor with short cytoplasmic tail; KIR-L: killer cell immunoglobulin-like receptor with long cytoplasmic tail; LAIR-1: leukocyte-associated immunoglobulin-like receptor 1; LILRB1: leukocyte immunoglobulin-like receptor B1; KLR: killer cell lectin-like receptor; NKR: NK cell receptor; SIGLEC: sialic acid-binding immunoglobulin-type lectins; HLA: human leukocyte antigen; LLT: lectin-like transcript 1. IgG: immunoglobulin G; BAT3: leukocyte antigen-B-associated transcript 3; MIC: MHC class I-related chain family; ULBP: UL16-binding proteins; HLA-G?: It is controversial whether HLA-G is a lignad of KIR2DL4.

Table 1.
NK cell receptors and their cognate ligands.

and they undergo apoptosis [16, 17]. Lastly, the cytokine pathway, NK cells secrete *various* cytokines, such as IFN-γ, TNF-α, GM-CSF and IL-10. These cytokines play an important role in immune responses of NK cells. For example, TNF-α alters the stability of lysosome in target cells, resulting in leakage of various hydrolases, effect on metabolism of cell membrane phospholipid and degradation of genomic DNA by endonuclease [18]. With these mechanisms, applications of NK cells have currently been established in tumor immunotherapy as chimeric antigen receptor-modified NK cells (CAR-NK cells) and adoptive immunotherapy.

3. *Killer immunoglobulin-like receptor (KIR)* polymorphisms mediated-heterogeneity of NK cell responses

Killer immunoglobulin-like receptors (KIRs) are cell surface receptors expressed on NK cells and subpopulation of T cells. Similar to HLA class I, KIR ligands, *KIRs* are highly polymorphic genes, including allelic polymorphisms, genes content and copy number variations [19]. Genetic variations of *KIRs* and *HLA* among individuals generate heterogeneity of immune responses of NK cells [20]. Interestingly, current evidences demonstrate the impact of *KIR* gene variations on disease susceptibility or resistance in several pathological conditions, such as infection, autoimmune/inflammatory disorder, implantation and particularly in hematopoietic stem cell transplantation [21]. Here, to better understand the role of NK cell alloreactivities, we thoroughly describe the basis of KIRs as well as its role in the immune system.

3.1 Killer immunoglobulin-like receptors (KIRs, CD158)

Killer immunoglobulin-like receptors are type I transmembrane glycoprotein expressed on the plasma membrane of NK cells, subpopulations of memory T cells and most of $CD8^+$ T cells [22, 23]. The KIR family consists of 15 functional genes (*KIR2DL1–4*, *2DL5A*, *2DL5B*, *2DS1–5*, *3DL1–3*, *3DS1*) and 2 pseudogenes (*2DP1* and *3DP1*) encoded within a 150 kb region of the leukocyte receptor complex (LRC) located on chromosome 19 (19q13.4) [24, 25] . The KIR proteins have either two or three extracellular immunoglobulin domains (KIR2D or KIR3D) and cytoplasmic (CYT) tails with long (L) or short (S) tails. Based on structural feature, a long *cytoplasmic tail* (KIR2DL or KIR3DL) contains immunoreceptor tyrosine-based inhibitory motif (ITIM) that functions to inhibit NK cell responses [26]. In contrast, a short *cytoplasmic tail* (KIR2DS or KIR3DS) has a positive charge amino acid residue in the transmembrane region to associate with DAP12 containing an immunoreceptor tyrosine-based activating motif (ITAM) that turns on NK cell functions [27]. Uniquely, KIR2DL4, a long cytoplasmic tail containing ITIM and linking with an adaptor molecule FcεRI, can deliver both activating and inhibitory signals to control NK cell responses [28, 29]. However, the mechanism by which KIR2DL4 delivers activating or inhibitory signals to NK cells is not established. Two pseudogenes, *KIR2DP1* and *KIR3DP1,* are not expressed on NK cells.

3.2 Diversity of *KIRs*

The extensive variation of *KIR* loci is achieved through allelic polymorphisms, a combination of gene content (absence/presence polymorphisms) and copy number variations. Firstly, allelic polymorphisms of *KIR* have been documented in the Immuno Polymorphism Database (IPD) showing each *KIR* locus contains 16–164 alleles of different genes [30]. Later, a combination of genes content generates distinct *KIR* genotypes, showing 625 different *KIR* genotypes reported in 171 populations worldwide [31]. Lastly, copy number variation (CNV) of *KIR* is currently studied and demonstrated that equal and unequal crossing over generates individual *KIR* gene duplication, deletion and hybridization [32]. Moreover, stochastic and variegated *KIR* expressions on NK cells by epigenetic regulation facilitate a diverse repertoire of NK cell clones within an individual [33] (**Figure 1**). As a consequence, the influence of *KIR* diversity on immune responses has been reported in several diseases [21, 34–36]. On the basis of gene content, *KIRs* are classified into group A and B haplotypes [37]. Both group A and B haplotypes are conserved with four framework genes (*KIR3DL3-3DP1-2DL4-3DL2*). Group A haplotype consists of the four framework genes and *2DL3*, *2DP1*, *2DL1*, *3DL1* or *2DS4*, whereas group B haplotype has variable gene content. Distinctly, group A haplotype shows predominantly inhibitory *KIR* genes except *KIR2DS4*, but group B haplotype contains dominantly activating *KIR* genes. The distributions of *KIR* haplotypes have been studied, showing variations of A and B are found among populations [38–43].

3.3 *KIR* and their cognate ligands

Both inhibitory and activating KIRs on NK cells recognize HLA class I molecules of target cells. Most KIR ligands have recently characterized as shown in **Table 2**, whereas some KIR ligands are still unknown [44–47]. The affinity of KIR and HLA interaction affects NK cell responses [48]. Remarkably, activating KIRs

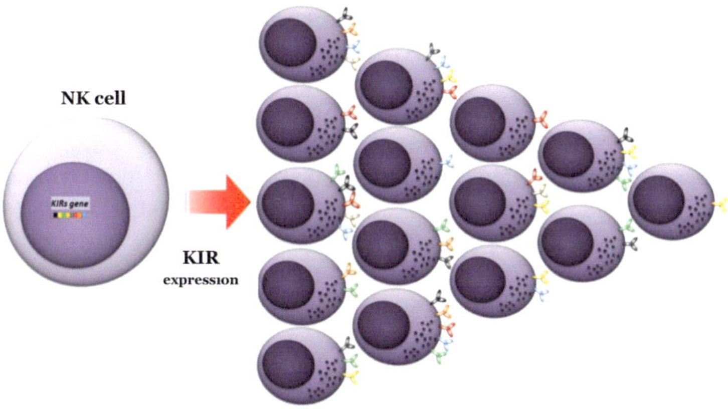

Figure 1.
NK cell repertoires. Individual KIR genotype generates a diverse repertoire of NK cells by stochastic expression. KIR expression on NK cells is influenced by HLA class I and CD94:NKG2A.

KIR	KIR ligand (HLA)	Function
2DL1	HLA-C2 (HLA-C^{Lys80})	Inhibition
2DL2	HLA-C1 (HLA-C^{Ans80})	Inhibition
2DL3	HLA-C1, HLA-C2 (weak)	Inhibition
2DL4	HLA-G?*	Activation/inhibition?
2DL5	Unknown	Inhibition
2DS1	HLA-C2 (HLA-C^{Lys80})	Activation
2DS2	HLA-C1 (HLA-C^{Ans80}), β_2-Microglobulin	Activation
2DS3	Unknown	Activation
2DS4	HLA-A11 and some HLA-C alleles	Activation
2DS5	Unknown	Inhibition
3DL1	HLA-Bw4	Inhibition
3DL2	HLA-A3, -A11	Inhibition
3DL3	Unknown	Inhibition
3DS1	HLA-Bw4?	Activation

The ligand for KIR2DL4 is still controversy [44, 45].

Table 2.
KIR and their ligands (HLA) specificity.

(KIR2DS1/2) and inhibitory KIRs (KIR2DL1/2) can bind the same HLA molecules. However, the affinity of inhibitory KIR-binding HLA is higher than activating KIR-binding HLA [49, 50]. It is believed that the lower affinity of activating KIR and HLA interaction would be evolved to avoid self-aggression.

4. Alloreactive NK cells from transplantation to adoptive immunotherapy

Over the past decade, adoptive transfer allogeneic NK cells have been emerged as promising immunotherapy for hematological malignancies [8, 51, 52]. The role of alloreactive NK cells is considered to be beneficial in achieving better outcomes after haploidentical HSCT (haplo-HSCT). Presently, haplo-HSCT is an alternative option when completely matched related or unrelated donors are not available. Historically, although haplo-HSCT can lead to graft versus host disease (GvHD) which has undesirable effect in post HSCT, this problem has been currently solved by performing of T cell depletion before graft infusion. After chemotherapy in AML patients, T cell prophylaxis has been used together with high stem cell doses, resulting in fast NK cell alloreactivities and slow T cell reconstitution. Moreover, graft versus leukemic cells mediated by NK cell, alloreactivities have been exploited which they can beneficially lead to reduced relapse, and improve survival [53]. Based on the interactions between NK cell receptors and their ligands, it was believed that allogeneic NK cells do not receive inhibition signals from the recipient HLA, leading NK cells to exert powerful anti-leukemia activity [54]. Regarding KIR-ligand mismatches between donor and recipient under haplo HSCT setting, alloreactive NK cells play crucial roles against leukemic cells, recipients' DCs and T cells [55], resulting in reduced leukemic relapses, GvHD and graft rejection, respectively (**Figure 2**). With these reasons, a number of studies have extensively investigated the role of KIR-ligand mismatches in both pre-clinical and clinical setting to evaluate the success in leukemia therapy. Additionally, four situations in predicting NK cell alloreactivities after haplo-HSCT have been proposed based on the deference in definition of KIR mismatches between the donor NK cells and the recipient's HLA [56] (**Figure 3**).

4.1 KIR-ligand (HLA) mismatch or missing-self-model

The KIR-ligand mismatch model, also called ligand incompatibility, has been proposed that an expression of HLA class I molecules (KIR ligand) on donor are

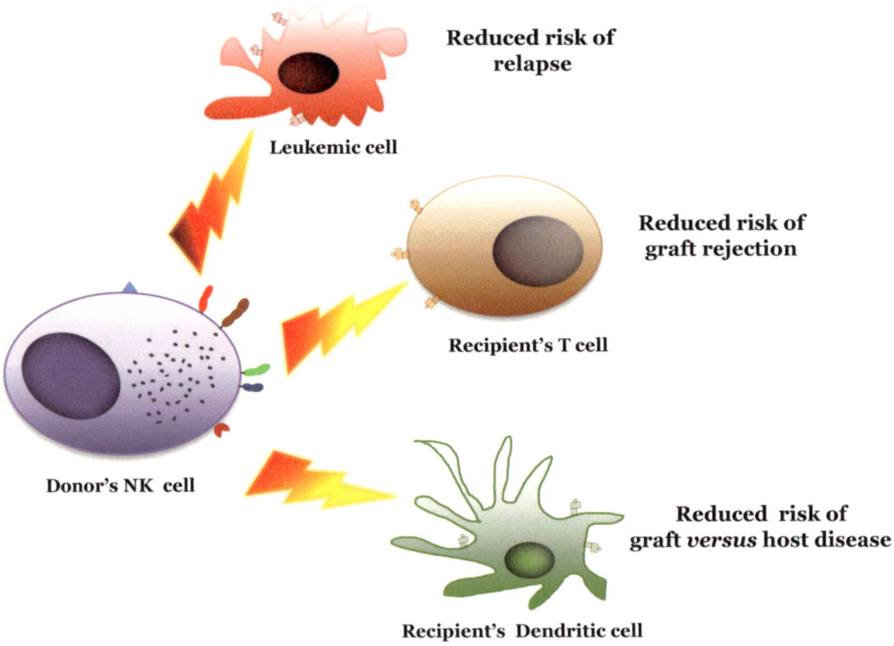

Figure 2.
The role of NK cell alloreactivities in acute leukemia. Beneficial effects of NK cell alloreactivities on the outcomes of acute leukemia under haplo-HSCT setting, adoptive transfer NK cells mediated activity against residual leukemic cells, recipient's T cells and dendritic cells, resulting in reduced the risk of relapse, graft rejection and GvHD, respectively.

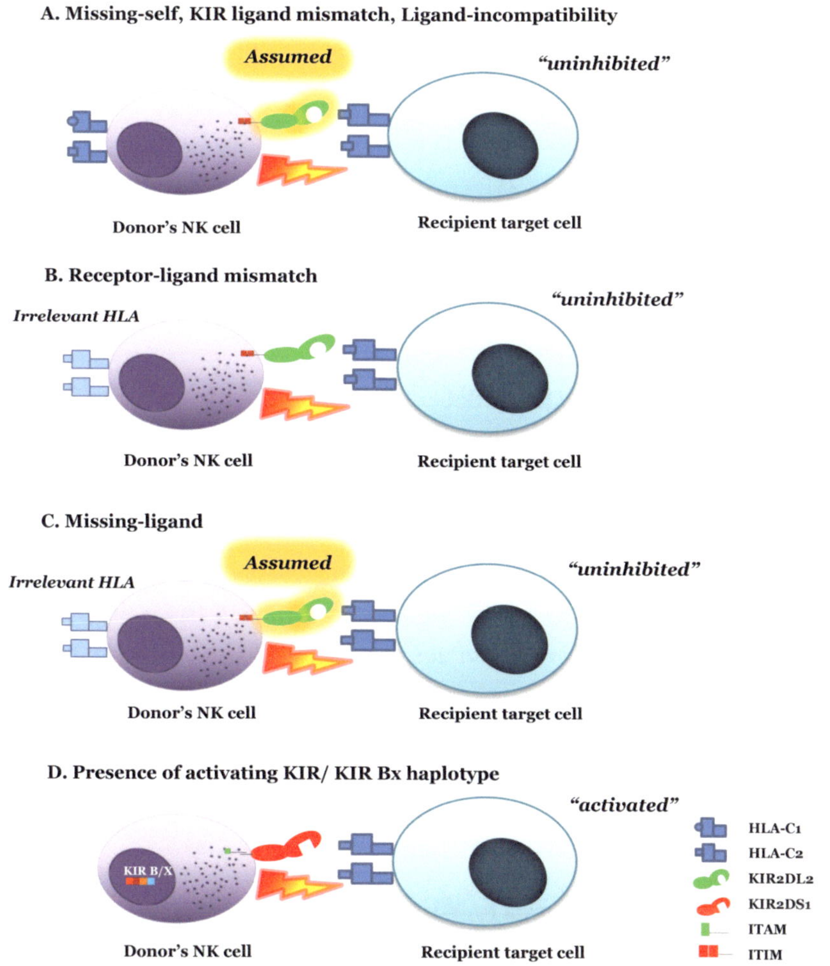

Figure 3.
Situations of NK cell alloreactivity in post-HSCT. (A) The KIR-ligand (HLA) mismatch or missing-self-model; NK cell alloreactivity is mediated by the lack of HLA ligand expression on recipient for inhibitory KIR on donor's NK cell which the presence of KIR expression on donor is assumed. High resolution HLA genotyping is performed in donor and recipient. (B) The receptor-ligand model; NK cell alloreactivity is mediated by the lack of HLA ligand expression on recipient for inhibitory KIR which the presence of KIR expression on donor NK cell is verified by genotyping and flow cytometry. The donor HLA is irrelevant to recipient. (C) The missing-ligand model; NK cell alloreactivity is mediated by the lack of at least one of HLA ligand (HLA-C1, -C2 or -Bw4) expression on recipient for inhibitory KIR and the donor HLA is irrelevant to recipient. (D) The presence of activating KIR model; NK cell alloreactivity is mediated by interaction of activating KIR on donor NK cell and HLA ligand on recipient target cell which KIR B haplotype contains more activating KIR than A/A haplotype. KIR genotyping was investigated in donor and recipient and some studies detected activating KIR on donor cells.

incompatible with recipient's HLA class I molecules [57, 58]. This model has been assumed that donor NK cells have inhibitory KIR that is missing its ligand on recipient. For example, NK cells from a HLA-C1/C2 donor will be alloreactive against a HLA-C2/C2 recipient, where it is assumed that KIR2DL2 is expressed on donor NK cells (**Figure 3A**).

4.2 Receptor-ligand mismatch model

The receptor-ligand mismatch model states that donor NK cells represent inhibitory KIR in mismatching with HLA class I on the recipient target cells, leading to NK cell alloreactivities in graft versus host direction [59]. This model is therefore required for KIR genotyping in donor as well as HLA typing in recipient (**Figure 3B**).

4.3 Missing-ligand model

Notably, the HLA is only genotyped in recipients and missing HLA-C1, C2 or Bw4 for inhibitory KIR on donor can lead to NK cell alloreactivities [58]. For example, recipient represents HLA-C2/C2, therefore, it is assumed (not investigated) that donor NK cells expressing KIR2DL2 to be alloreactive due to missing HLA-C1 ligand (**Figure 3C**).

4.4 Presence of activating KIR model

Here, in this model, activating KIR on donor cells is measured to predict NK cell alloreactivities because the interactions between donor activating KIRs and their ligands on recipient can lead to NK cells achieving activation signals [60] (**Figure 3D**).

5. The role of NK cell alloreactivities in post HSCT

Several studies have revealed an influence of alloreactive NK cells in acute leukemia patients, where alloreactive NK cells deliver promising better outcomes in term of anti-leukemia activity. Predominantly, KIR-mediated NK alloreactivity has been demonstrated to be the most clinically significant relevance to AML, while its role in ALL remains unclear.

5.1 Acute myeloblastic leukemia (AML)

As acute myeloblastic leukemia was more susceptible to NK cell cytotoxicity than solid tumors [61], the role of adoptive transfer NK cells against leukemia was investigated in AML patients [62]. Anti-leukemic effect of allogeneic NK cells has been extensively studied under haplo-HSCT with the mismatches of KIR and cognate ligands between donor and recipient. Interestingly, Ruggeri and coworkers initially reported allogeneic NK cells mediated cytotoxicity against recipients' leukemic cells [53]. Later, the impact of NK cells alloreactivity in preventing AML relapse, GVHD and rejection was confirmed in clinical setting and mouse model [63]. Taken together, this condition has been explored under T cell depleted to avoid graft versus host effect and high doses of infused stem cell transplantation [54, 63, 64]. Remarkably, this approach was investigated in 21 AML children who received haplo-HSCT, showing donor-derived alloreactive NK cells killed leukemic cells in KIR-ligand mismatches, even late after transplantation [7]. Altogether, the doses of infused NK cell and immunosuppression were evaluated in children with AML to consider safety and effectiveness of alloreactive NK cells therapy [65]. Moreover, successfully transferred NK cells immunotherapy were reported in elderly AML who were not candidates for HSCT, demonstrating this approach was feasible and safe in elderly patients [8, 66].

Haplo-HSCT with KIR-ligand mismatches has been a promising strategy in AML for adoptive transfer of NK cells for immunotherapy [67, 68]. The incompatibility of three main inhibitory *KIR* loci (*2DL1*, *2DL2/3* and *3DL1*) with their ligands (*HLA-C2*, *HLA-C1* and *HLA-Bw4*) has been extensively investigated, and found to be relevant for better clinical outcomes [69, 70]. To explain the potential benefits of alloreactive NK cells against leukemia based on an absence of inhibitory signal delivered by KIR on donor's NK cells, it has been shown that KIR2DL1$^+$ NK cells lyse leukemia in HLA-C1/C1 recipients, whereas KIR2DL2/3$^+$ NK cells partially lyse leukemia in HLA-C2/C2 recipients due to low-affinity binding, and that KIR3DL1 + NK cells lyse HLA-Bw4$^-$ leukemia of recipients, where HLA-Bw4$^-$ would be HLA-A or HLA-B as determined by the serotypic specificity. However, for the activating KIR model, KIR2DS1$^+$NK cells have demonstrated a potent reactivity against HLA-C2 expressing allogeneic target cells *in vitro* [60, 71], particularly on T cells and dendritic cells. As mentioned, although NK cell-based immunotherapy has been a promising approach in adult and childhood [8, 65, 66], there are additional issues that need to be considered in achieving a successful therapy. Firstly, the minimum or optimal number of infused NK cells is really required to achieve therapeutic effect that remains inconclusive due to lack of standardized technical procedure for qualifying alloreactive NK cells [67, 68]. Additionally, it became clear that infused NK cells favor IL-2 and IL-15 for expansion and survival [51, 72], however, administration of IL-15 after infusion has been recommended because IL-2 can promote host regulatory T cells to inhibit allogeneic NK cells.

Given the crucial role of alloreactive NK cells in graft versus leukemia (GVL) effect in haplo-HSCT, the predictive algorithm for donor selection is being developed in AML treatment. Several research groups have explored feasibility of NK cell-based immunotherapy, including *in vivo* and *in vitro* studies as well as clinical trials. Predominantly, mismatches of donors' inhibitory KIR expressing NK cells (2DL1, KIR2DL2/3 and KIR3DL1) with HLA class I of the patients have been well-documented that were relevant to therapeutic effect of NK immunotherapy in AML [7, 66, 73]. For activating KIRs, only KIR2DS1 has been reported to associate with NK cell alloreactivities against target cells expressing HLA-C2 [60, 74]. Moreover, *KIR* haplotypes and clinical outcomes have been observed, showing donors with group B *KIR* haplotype have improved relapse—free survival for AML patients under unrelated HSCT [75]. With these reasons, KIR-mediated NK cell functions in haplo-HSCT should be taken in to account for donor selections, since the potential benefit of NK alloreactivity has improved survival and clinical outcomes in AML patients. Moreover, phase I and II clinical trials have been being studied to evaluate the feasibility and safety [76, 77] for further applications. Therefore, haplo-HSCT with T cell depletion, KIR-mediated NK cell alloreactivities should be considered for donor selections using an algorithm in which KIR-ligand mismatches could be predicted. This is available as an online calculator (https://www.ebi.ac.uk/ipd/kir/ligand.html).

5.2 Acute lymphoblastic leukemia (ALL)

Since the role of alloreactive NK cells in AML were reported, the influence of KIR on the outcome of ALL patients in haplo-HSCT setting has been investigated. Like AML, the approach based upon KIR-ligand mismatches and the presence of donor's KIR2DS1$^+$ NK cells with HLA-C2 expressing target cells mediated NK cell alloreactivities against leukemic blasts has been tested [7]. In addition, ALL children transplanted from a *KIR* haplotype B donor showed significantly reduced risk of relapse, particularly in donors with high B content score [78]. However, the beneficial effect of NK cell alloreactivity has not been obviously noticeable in ALL patients in particular mechanisms of NK cells against ALL tumor cells [63, 79, 80]. The clinical studies of beneficial effect of NK cell alloreactivities in acute leukemia are summarized in **Table 3**.

Study	Disease	Model	Beneficial effect	Ref.
Ruggeri et al. (1999)	AML, ALL, CML	KIR-ligand mismatch	Antileukemic effect	[53]
Ruggeri et al. (2002)	AML, ALL	KIR-ligand mismatch	Reduced relapse, Reduces graft rejection, protected GvHD	[63]
Miller et al. (2007)	AML, MDS, CML	Missing-ligand	Reduced relapse	[81]
Pende et al. (2008)	AML, ALL	KIR-ligand mismatch	Antileukemic effect	[7]
Rubnitz et al. (2009)	AML	Receptor-ligand mismatch	No GvHD	[65]
Willemze et al. (2009)	AML, ALL	KIR-ligand mismatch	Reduced relapse	[82]
Cooley et al. (2009)	AML	KIR haplotype, KIR-ligand mismatch	Improved survival rate	[75]
Cooley et al. (2010)	AML, ALL	KIR haplotype	Reduced relapse	[83]
Venstrom et al. (2010)	AML, MDS, CML, ALL	KIR haplotype	Decreased acute GvHD	[84]
Curti et al. (2011)	AML	KIR-ligand mismatch	Antileukemic effect	[8]
Venstrom et al. (2012)	AML	Missing-ligand, receptor-ligand mismatch, presence of activating *KIR*	KIR2DS1 associated with lower relapse, KIR3DS1 associated with lower mortality	[74]
Cooley et al. (2014)	AML	Missing-ligand, KIR haplotype	Reduced relapse	[85]
Curti et al. (2016)	AML	KIR-ligand mismatch	Reduced relapse	[66]

AML: acute myeloid leukemia; ALL, acute lymphoid leukemia; CML: chronic myeloid leukemia; MDS: myelodysplastic syndromes; GvHD: graft versus host disease.

Table 3.
Clinical studies of beneficial effects of NK cell alloreactivities in acute leukemia.

6. Conclusion

This chapter sheds light on adoptive transfer NK cell immunotherapy in haplo-HSCT setting after immunosuppressive chemotherapy. KIR-ligand mismatches, activating KIR with cognate ligand as well as *KIR* B haplotype, could contribute to the potential benefit of allogeneic NK cells against acute leukemia in improving relapse-free and survival in AML patients. Additionally, the donor selection algorithm based on KIR-ligand mismatches is provided and available. Conflicts resulted from studies could be explained by the different definitions of KIR ligand mismatches, failure of infused NK cells to expand and persist, extensive genetic polymorphisms as well as the stochastic surface expressions of specific KIRs on individual NK cells. However, some limitations still need to be elucidated in further studies to overcome obstacles and achieve successful NK cell immunotherapy and clinical impact. For example, the ligands for KIR2DL5 and KIR2DS3 are still unknown. In addition, the molecular mechanisms of KIR and NK cells need to be well-established. Eventually, this chapter provides a promising approach of NK cell-based immunotherapy that has revolutionized hematologic malignancy treatment, particularly AML, however, the feasibility has been challenged by complexity and understanding of NK cell biology as well as KIRs.

Acknowledgements

SC was supported by Thailand Research Fund and the Commission on Higher Education under the Grant for New Researcher (No. MRG6180172).

Conflict of interest

The authors declare no conflict of interest.

Author details

Suwit Chaisri[1*] and Chanvit Leelayuwat[2]

1 Chulabhorn International College of Medicine (CICM), Thammasat University, Pathum Thani, Thailand

2 The Centre for Research and Development of Medical Diagnostic Laboratories (CMDL), Department of Clinical Immunology and Transfusion Sciences, Faculty of Associated Medical Sciences, Khon Kaen University, Khon Kaen, Thailand

*Address all correspondence to: chaisrisuw@gmail.com

IntechOpen

© 2019 The Author(s). Licensee IntechOpen. This chapter is distributed under the terms of the Creative Commons Attribution License (http://creativecommons.org/licenses/by/3.0), which permits unrestricted use, distribution, and reproduction in any medium, provided the original work is properly cited.

References

[1] Rezvani K, Rouce RH. The application of natural killer cell immunotherapy for the treatment of cancer. Frontiers in Immunology. 2015;**6**:578. DOI: 10.3389/fimmu.2015.00578

[2] Paul S, Lal G. The molecular mechanism of natural killer cells function and its importance in cancer immunotherapy. Frontiers in Immunology. 2017;**8**:1124. DOI: 10.3389/fimmu.2017.01124

[3] Zhang J, Zheng H, Diao Y. Natural killer cells and current applications of chimeric antigen receptor-modified NK-92 cells in tumor immunotherapy. International Journal of Molecular Sciences. 2019;**20**(2):317. DOI: 10.3390/ijms20020317

[4] Rezvani K, Rouce R, Liu E, Shpall E. Engineering natural killer cells for cancer immunotherapy. Molecular Therapy. 2017;**25**(8):1769-1781. DOI: 10.1016/j.ymthe.2017.06.012

[5] Mehta RS, Randolph B, Daher M, Rezvani K. NK cell therapy for hematologic malignancies. International Journal of Hematology. 2018;**107**(3):262-270. DOI: 10.1007/s12185-018-2407-5

[6] Handgretinger R, Lang P, Andre MC. Exploitation of natural killer cells for the treatment of acute leukemia. Blood. 2016;**127**(26):3341-3349. DOI: 10.1182/blood-2015-12-629055

[7] Pende D, Marcenaro S, Falco M, Martini S, Bernardo ME, Montagna D, et al. Anti-leukemia activity of alloreactive NK cells in KIR ligand-mismatched haploidentical HSCT for pediatric patients: Evaluation of the functional role of activating KIR and redefinition of inhibitory KIR specificity. Blood. 2009;**113**(13):3119-3129. DOI: 10.1182/blood-2008-06-164103

[8] Curti A, Ruggeri L, D'Addio A, Bontadini A, Dan E, Motta MR, et al. Successful transfer of alloreactive haploidentical KIR ligand-mismatched natural killer cells after infusion in elderly high risk acute myeloid leukemia patients. Blood. 2011;**118**(12):3273-3279. DOI: 10.1182/blood-2011-01-329508

[9] Cerwenka A, Lanier LL. Natural killer cell memory in infection, inflammation and cancer. Nature Reviews. Immunology. 2016;**16**(2):112-123. DOI: 10.1038/nri.2015.9

[10] Hammer Q, Ruckert T, Romagnani C. Natural killer cell specificity for viral infections. Nature Immunology. 2018;**19**(8):800-808. DOI: 10.1038/s41590-018-0163-6

[11] Vivier E, Tomasello E, Baratin M, Walzer T, Ugolini S. Functions of natural killer cells. Nature Immunology. 2008;**9**(5):503-510. DOI: 10.1038/ni1582

[12] Vivier E, Nunes JA, Vely F. Natural killer cell signaling pathways. Science. 2004;**306**(5701):1517-1519. DOI: 10.1126/science.1103478

[13] Long EO, Kim HS, Liu D, Peterson ME, Rajagopalan S. Controlling natural killer cell responses: Integration of signals for activation and inhibition. Annual Review of Immunology. 2013;**31**:227-258. DOI: 10.1146/annurev-immunol-020711-075005

[14] Kim S, Poursine-Laurent J, Truscott SM, Lybarger L, Song YJ, Yang L, et al. Licensing of natural killer cells by host major histocompatibility complex class I molecules. Nature. 2005;**436**(7051):709-713. DOI: 10.1038/nature03847

[15] Topham NJ, Hewitt EW. Natural killer cell cytotoxicity: How do they pull the trigger? Immunology. 2009;**128**(1):7-15. DOI: 10.1111/j.1365-2567.2009.03123.x

[16] Mercer F, Kozhaya L, Unutmaz D. Expression and function of TNF and IL-1 receptors on human regulatory T cells. PLoS One. 2010;**5**(1):e8639. DOI: 10.1371/journal.pone.0008639

[17] Wajant H. The Fas signaling pathway: More than a paradigm. Science. 2002;**296**(5573):1635-1636. DOI: 10.1126/science.1071553

[18] Chiossone L, Dumas PY, Vienne M, Vivier E. Natural killer cells and other innate lymphoid cells in cancer. Nature Reviews. Immunology. 2018;**18**(11): 671-688. DOI: 10.1038/s41577-018-0061-z

[19] Chaisri S, Traherne JA, Jayaraman J, Romphruk A, Trowsdale J, Leelayuwat C. Novel KIR genotypes and gene copy number variations in northeastern Thais. Immunology. 2018;**153**(3): 380-386. DOI: 10.1111/imm.12847

[20] Yawata M, Yawata N, Draghi M, Little AM, Partheniou F, Parham P. Roles for HLA and KIR polymorphisms in natural killer cell repertoire selection and modulation of effector function. The Journal of Experimental Medicine. 2006;**203**(3):633-645. DOI: 10.1084/jem.20051884

[21] Kulkarni S, Martin MP, Carrington M. The Yin and Yang of HLA and KIR in human disease. Seminars in Immunology. 2008;**20**(6):343-352. DOI: 10.1016/j.smim.2008.06.003

[22] Bakker AB, Phillips JH, Figdor CG, Lanier LL. Killer cell inhibitory receptors for MHC class I molecules regulate lysis of melanoma cells mediated by NK cells, gamma delta T cells, and antigen-specific CTL. Journal of Immunology. 1998;**160**(11):5239-5245. Epub 1998/05/30

[23] Mingari MC, Ponte M, Vitale C, Bellomo R, Moretta L. Expression of HLA class I-specific inhibitory receptors in human cytolytic T lymphocytes: A regulated mechanism that controls T-cell activation and function. Human Immunology. 2000;**61**(1):44-50. Epub 2000/02/05. DOI: S0198-8859(99)00158-5 [pii]

[24] Trowsdale J, Barten R, Haude A, Stewart CA, Beck S, Wilson MJ. The genomic context of natural killer receptor extended gene families. Immunological Reviews. 2001;**181**: 20-38. Epub 2001/08/22

[25] Wende H, Colonna M, Ziegler A, Volz A. Organization of the leukocyte receptor cluster (LRC) on human chromosome 19q13.4. Mammalian Genome. 1999;**10**(2):154-160. Epub 1999/01/29

[26] Hsu KC, Chida S, Geraghty DE, Dupont B. The killer cell immunoglobulin-like receptor (KIR) genomic region: Gene-order, haplotypes and allelic polymorphism. Immunological Reviews. 2002;**190**: 40-52. Epub 2002/12/21

[27] Lanier LL, Corliss BC, Wu J, Leong C, Phillips JH. Immunoreceptor DAP12 bearing a tyrosine-based activation motif is involved in activating NK cells. Nature. 1998;**391**(6668):703-707. Epub 1998/03/07. DOI: 10.1038/35642

[28] Rajagopalan S, Moyle MW, Joosten I, Long EO. DNA-PKcs controls an endosomal signaling pathway for a proinflammatory response by natural killer cells. Science Signaling. 2010;**3**(110):ra14. Epub 2010/02/25. DOI: 10.1126/scisignal.2000467

[29] Faure M, Long EO. KIR2DL4 (CD158d), an NK cell-activating receptor with inhibitory potential. Journal of Immunology. 2002;**168**(12):6208-6214. Epub 2002/06/11

[30] Robinson J, Halliwell JA, McWilliam H, Lopez R, Marsh SG.

IPD—The Immuno Polymorphism Database. Nucleic Acids Research. 2013;**41**(Database issue):D1234-D1240. Epub 2012/11/28. DOI: 10.1093/nar/gks1140

[31] Gonzalez-Galarza FF, Takeshita LY, Santos EJ, Kempson F, Maia MH, da Silva AL, et al. Allele frequency net 2015 update: New features for HLA epitopes, KIR and disease and HLA adverse drug reaction associations. Nucleic Acids Research. 2015;**43**(Database issue):D784-D788. Epub 2014/11/22. DOI: 10.1093/nar/gku1166

[32] Pyo CW, Guethlein LA, Vu Q, Wang R, Abi-Rached L, Norman PJ, et al. Different patterns of evolution in the centromeric and telomeric regions of group A and B haplotypes of the human killer cell Ig-like receptor locus. PLoS One. 2010;**5**(12):e15115. Epub 2011/01/06. DOI: 10.1371/journal.pone.0015115

[33] Shilling HG, Young N, Guethlein LA, Cheng NW, Gardiner CM, Tyan D, et al. Genetic control of human NK cell repertoire. Journal of Immunology. 2002;**169**(1):239-247

[34] Williams AP, Bateman AR, Khakoo SI. Hanging in the balance. KIR and their role in disease. Molecular Interventions. 2005;**5**(4):226-240. Epub 2005/08/27. DOI: 10.1124/mi.5.4.6

[35] Bashirova AA, Martin MP, McVicar DW, Carrington M. The killer immunoglobulin-like receptor gene cluster: Tuning the genome for defense. Annual Review of Genomics and Human Genetics. 2006;7:277-300. Epub 2006/07/11. DOI: 10.1146/annurev.genom.7.080505.115726

[36] Takeshita LY, Gonzalez-Galarza FF, dos Santos EJ, Maia MH, Rahman MM, Zain SM, et al. A database for curating the associations between killer cell immunoglobulin-like receptors and diseases in worldwide populations. Database: The Journal of Biological Databases and Curation. 2013;**2013**:bat021. Epub 2013/04/16. DOI: 10.1093/database/bat021

[37] Uhrberg M, Valiante NM, Shum BP, Shilling HG, Lienert-Weidenbach K, Corliss B, et al. Human diversity in killer cell inhibitory receptor genes. Immunity. 1997;**7**(6):753-763. Epub 1998/01/16. DOI: S1074-7613(00)80394-5 [pii]

[38] Toneva M, Lepage V, Lafay G, Dulphy N, Busson M, Lester S, et al. Genomic diversity of natural killer cell receptor genes in three populations. Tissue Antigens. 2001;**57**(4):358-362. Epub 2001/07/14. DOI: tan570411 [pii]

[39] Norman PJ, Stephens HA, Verity DH, Chandanayingyong D, Vaughan RW. Distribution of natural killer cell immunoglobulin-like receptor sequences in three ethnic groups. Immunogenetics. 2001;**52**(3-4):195-205. Epub 2001/02/28

[40] Rajalingam R, Du Z, Meenagh A, Luo L, Kavitha VJ, Pavithra-Arulvani R, et al. Distinct diversity of KIR genes in three southern Indian populations: Comparison with world populations revealed a link between KIR gene content and pre-historic human migrations. Immunogenetics. 2008;**60**(5):207-217. Epub 2008/03/29. DOI: 10.1007/s00251-008-0286-2

[41] Wu GQ, Zhao YM, Lai XY, Yang KL, Zhu FM, Zhang W, et al. Distribution of killer-cell immunoglobulin-like receptor genes in Eastern mainland Chinese Han and Taiwanese Han populations. Tissue Antigens. 2009;**74**(6):499-507. Epub 2009/09/19. DOI: 10.1111/j.1399-0039.2009.01366.x

[42] Rajalingam R, Krausa P, Shilling HG, Stein JB, Balamurugan A, McGinnis MD, et al. Distinctive KIR and HLA diversity in a panel of north Indian Hindus. Immunogenetics. 2002;**53**(12):

1009-1019. Epub 2002/03/21. DOI: 10.1007/s00251-001-0425-5

[43] Chaisri S, Kitcharoen K, Romphruk AV, Romphruk A, Witt CS, Leelayuwat C. Polymorphisms of killer immunoglobulin-like receptors (KIRs) and HLA ligands in northeastern Thais. Immunogenetics. 2013;**65**(9):645-653. Epub 2013/07/03. DOI: 10.1007/s00251-013-0716-7

[44] Moradi S, Berry R, Pymm P, Hitchen C, Beckham SA, Wilce MC, et al. The structure of the atypical killer cell immunoglobulin-like receptor, KIR2DL4. The Journal of Biological Chemistry. 2015;**290**(16):10460-10471. DOI: 10.1074/jbc.M114.612291

[45] Le Page ME, Goodridge JP, John E, Christiansen FT, Witt CS. Response to comment on "killer Ig-like receptor 2DL4 does not mediate NK cell IFN-gamma responses to soluble HLA-G preparations". Journal of Immunology. 2014;**192**(9):4003-4004. DOI: 10.4049/jimmunol.1400492

[46] Jamil KM, Khakoo SI. KIR/HLA interactions and pathogen immunity. Journal of Biomedicine & Biotechnology. 2011;**2011**:298348. Epub 2011/06/02. DOI: 10.1155/2011/298348

[47] Thiruchelvam-Kyle L, Hoelsbrekken SE, Saether PC, Bjornsen EG, Pende D, Fossum S, et al. The activating human NK cell receptor KIR2DS2 recognizes a beta2-microglobulin-independent ligand on cancer cells. Journal of Immunology. 2017;**198**(7):2556-2567. DOI: 10.4049/jimmunol.1600930

[48] Purdy AK, Campbell KS. Natural killer cells and cancer: Regulation by the killer cell Ig-like receptors (KIR). Cancer Biology & Therapy. 2009;**8**(23):2211-2220. Epub 2009/11/20

[49] Biassoni R, Pessino A, Malaspina A, Cantoni C, Bottino C, Sivori S, et al. Role of amino acid position 70 in the binding affinity of p50.1 and p58.1 receptors for HLA-Cw4 molecules. European Journal of Immunology. 1997;**27**(12):3095-3099. Epub 1998/02/17. DOI: 10.1002/eji.1830271203

[50] Vales-Gomez M, Erskine RA, Deacon MP, Strominger JL, Reyburn HT. The role of zinc in the binding of killer cell Ig-like receptors to class I MHC proteins. Proceedings of the National Academy of Sciences of the United States of America. 2001;**98**(4):1734-1739. Epub 2001/02/15. DOI: 10.1073/pnas.041618298

[51] Miller JS, Soignier Y, Panoskaltsis-Mortari A, McNearney SA, Yun GH, Fautsch SK, et al. Successful adoptive transfer and in vivo expansion of human haploidentical NK cells in patients with cancer. Blood. 2005;**105**(8):3051-3057. DOI: 10.1182/blood-2004-07-2974

[52] Rodriguez NA, Meier PP, Groer MW, Zeller JM, Engstrom JL, Fogg L. A pilot study to determine the safety and feasibility of oropharyngeal administration of own mother's colostrum to extremely low-birth-weight infants. Advances in Neonatal Care. 2010;**10**(4):206-212. DOI: 10.1097/ANC.0b013e3181e94133

[53] Ruggeri L, Capanni M, Casucci M, Volpi I, Tosti A, Perruccio K, et al. Role of natural killer cell alloreactivity in HLA-mismatched hematopoietic stem cell transplantation. Blood. 1999;**94**(1):333-339

[54] Aversa F, Tabilio A, Terenzi A, Velardi A, Falzetti F, Giannoni C, et al. Successful engraftment of T-cell-depleted haploidentical "three-loci" incompatible transplants in leukemia patients by addition of recombinant human granulocyte colony-stimulating factor-mobilized peripheral blood progenitor cells to bone marrow inoculum. Blood. 1994;**84**(11):3948-3955

[55] Locatelli F, Pende D, Mingari MC, Bertaina A, Falco M, Moretta A, et al. Cellular and molecular basis of haploidentical hematopoietic stem cell transplantation in the successful treatment of high-risk leukemias: Role of alloreactive NK cells. Frontiers in Immunology. 2013;**4**:15. DOI: 10.3389/fimmu.2013.00015

[56] Heidenreich S, Kroger N. Reduction of relapse after unrelated donor stem cell transplantation by KIR-based graft selection. Frontiers in Immunology. 2017;**8**:41. DOI: 10.3389/fimmu.2017.00041

[57] Ljunggren HG, Karre K. In search of the 'missing self': MHC molecules and NK cell recognition. Immunology Today. 1990;**11**(7):237-244

[58] Symons HJ, Fuchs EJ. Hematopoietic SCT from partially HLA-mismatched (HLA-haploidentical) related donors. Bone Marrow Transplantation. 2008;**42**(6):365-377. DOI: 10.1038/bmt.2008.215

[59] Ruggeri L, Mancusi A, Capanni M, Urbani E, Carotti A, Aloisi T, et al. Donor natural killer cell allorecognition of missing self in haploidentical hematopoietic transplantation for acute myeloid leukemia: Challenging its predictive value. Blood. 2007;**110**(1):433-440. DOI: 10.1182/blood-2006-07-038687

[60] Chewning JH, Gudme CN, Hsu KC, Selvakumar A, Dupont B. KIR2DS1-positive NK cells mediate alloresponse against the C2 HLA-KIR ligand group in vitro. Journal of Immunology. 2007;**179**(2):854-868

[61] Guillerey C, Huntington ND, Smyth MJ. Targeting natural killer cells in cancer immunotherapy. Nature Immunology. 2016;**17**(9):1025-1036. DOI: 10.1038/ni.3518

[62] Ruggeri L, Parisi S, Urbani E, Curti A. Alloreactive natural killer cells for the treatment of acute myeloid leukemia: From stem cell transplantation to adoptive immunotherapy. Frontiers in Immunology. 2015;**6**:479. DOI: 10.3389/fimmu.2015.00479

[63] Ruggeri L, Capanni M, Urbani E, Perruccio K, Shlomchik WD, Tosti A, et al. Effectiveness of donor natural killer cell alloreactivity in mismatched hematopoietic transplants. Science. 2002;**295**(5562):2097-2100. DOI: 10.1126/science.1068440

[64] Koehl U, Sorensen J, Esser R, Zimmermann S, Gruttner HP, Tonn T, et al. IL-2 activated NK cell immunotherapy of three children after haploidentical stem cell transplantation. Blood Cells, Molecules & Diseases. 2004;**33**(3):261-266. DOI: 10.1016/j.bcmd.2004.08.013

[65] Rubnitz JE, Inaba H, Ribeiro RC, Pounds S, Rooney B, Bell T, et al. NKAML: A pilot study to determine the safety and feasibility of haploidentical natural killer cell transplantation in childhood acute myeloid leukemia. Journal of Clinical Oncology. 2010;**28**(6):955-959. DOI: 10.1200/JCO.2009.24.4590

[66] Curti A, Ruggeri L, Parisi S, Bontadini A, Dan E, Motta MR, et al. Larger size of donor alloreactive NK cell repertoire correlates with better response to NK cell immunotherapy in elderly acute myeloid leukemia patients. Clinical Cancer Research. 2016;**22**(8):1914-1921. DOI: 10.1158/1078-0432.CCR-15-1604

[67] Parisi S, Lecciso M, Ocadlikova D, Salvestrini V, Ciciarello M, Forte D, et al. The more, the better: "Do the right thing" for natural killer immunotherapy in acute myeloid leukemia. Frontiers in Immunology. 2017;**8**:1330. DOI: 10.3389/fimmu.2017.01330

[68] Muntasell A, Lopez-Botet M. Natural killer cell-based immunotherapy

in acute myeloid leukemia: Lessons for the future. Clinical Cancer Research. 2016;**22**(8):1831-1833. DOI: 10.1158/1078-0432.CCR-15-3168

[69] Giebel S, Locatelli F, Lamparelli T, Velardi A, Davies S, Frumento G, et al. Survival advantage with KIR ligand incompatibility in hematopoietic stem cell transplantation from unrelated donors. Blood. 2003;**102**(3):814-819. DOI: 10.1182/blood-2003-01-0091

[70] Hsu KC, Gooley T, Malkki M, Pinto-Agnello C, Dupont B, Bignon JD, et al. KIR ligands and prediction of relapse after unrelated donor hematopoietic cell transplantation for hematologic malignancy. Biology of Blood and Marrow Transplantation. 2006;**12**(8):828-836. DOI: 10.1016/j.bbmt.2006.04.008

[71] Sivori S, Carlomagno S, Falco M, Romeo E, Moretta L, Moretta A. Natural killer cells expressing the KIR2DS1-activating receptor efficiently kill T-cell blasts and dendritic cells: Implications in haploidentical HSCT. Blood. 2011;**117**(16):4284-4292. DOI: 10.1182/blood-2010-10-316125

[72] Bachanova V, Cooley S, Defor TE, Verneris MR, Zhang B, McKenna DH, et al. Clearance of acute myeloid leukemia by haploidentical natural killer cells is improved using IL-2 diphtheria toxin fusion protein. Blood. 2014;**123**(25):3855-3863. DOI: 10.1182/blood-2013-10-532531

[73] Boudreau JE, Giglio F, Gooley TA, Stevenson PA, Le Luduec JB, Shaffer BC, et al. KIR3DL1/HL A-B subtypes govern acute myelogenous leukemia relapse after hematopoietic cell transplantation. Journal of Clinical Oncology. 2017;**35**(20):2268-2278. DOI: 10.1200/JCO.2016.70.7059

[74] Venstrom JM, Pittari G, Gooley TA, Chewning JH, Spellman S, Haagenson M, et al. HLA-C-dependent prevention of leukemia relapse by donor activating KIR2DS1. The New England Journal of Medicine. 2012;**367**(9):805-816. DOI: 10.1056/NEJMoa1200503

[75] Cooley S, Trachtenberg E, Bergemann TL, Saeteurn K, Klein J, Le CT, et al. Donors with group B KIR haplotypes improve relapse-free survival after unrelated hematopoietic cell transplantation for acute myelogenous leukemia. Blood. 2009;**113**(3):726-732. DOI: 10.1182/blood-2008-07-171926

[76] Shaffer BC, Le Luduec JB, Forlenza C, Jakubowski AA, Perales MA, Young JW, et al. Phase II study of haploidentical natural killer cell infusion for treatment of relapsed or persistent myeloid malignancies following allogeneic hematopoietic cell transplantation. Biology of Blood and Marrow Transplantation. 2016;**22**(4):705-709. DOI: 10.1016/j.bbmt.2015.12.028

[77] Lee DA, Denman CJ, Rondon G, Woodworth G, Chen J, Fisher T, et al. Haploidentical natural killer cells infused before allogeneic stem cell transplantation for myeloid malignancies: A phase I trial. Biology of Blood and Marrow Transplantation. 2016;**22**(7):1290-1298. DOI: 10.1016/j.bbmt.2016.04.009

[78] Oevermann L, Michaelis SU, Mezger M, Lang P, Toporski J, Bertaina A, et al. KIR B haplotype donors confer a reduced risk for relapse after haploidentical transplantation in children with ALL. Blood. 2014;**124**(17):2744-2747. DOI: 10.1182/blood-2014-03-565069

[79] Brentjens RJ. Cellular therapies in acute lymphoblastic leukemia. Current Opinion in Molecular Therapeutics. 2009;**11**(4):375-382

[80] Romanski A, Bug G, Becker S, Kampfmann M, Seifried E, Hoelzer D, et al. Mechanisms of resistance to natural killer cell-mediated

cytotoxicity in acute lymphoblastic leukemia. Experimental Hematology. 2005;**33**(3):344-352. DOI: 10.1016/j.exphem.2004.11.006

[81] Miller JS, Cooley S, Parham P, Farag SS, Verneris MR, McQueen KL, et al. Missing KIR ligands are associated with less relapse and increased graft-versus-host disease (GVHD) following unrelated donor allogeneic HCT. Blood. 2007;**109**(11):5058-5061. DOI: 10.1182/blood-2007-01-065383

[82] Willemze R, Rodrigues CA, Labopin M, Sanz G, Michel G, Socie G, et al. KIR-ligand incompatibility in the graft-versus-host direction improves outcomes after umbilical cord blood transplantation for acute leukemia. Leukemia. 2009;**23**(3):492-500. DOI: 10.1038/leu.2008.365

[83] Cooley S, Weisdorf DJ, Guethlein LA, Klein JP, Wang T, Le CT, et al. Donor selection for natural killer cell receptor genes leads to superior survival after unrelated transplantation for acute myelogenous leukemia. Blood. 2010;**116**(14):2411-2419. DOI: 10.1182/blood-2010-05-283051

[84] Venstrom JM, Gooley TA, Spellman S, Pring J, Malkki M, Dupont B, et al. Donor activating KIR3DS1 is associated with decreased acute GVHD in unrelated allogeneic hematopoietic stem cell transplantation. Blood. 2010;**115**(15):3162-3165. DOI: 10.1182/blood-2009-08-236943

[85] Cooley S, Weisdorf DJ, Guethlein LA, Klein JP, Wang T, Marsh SG, et al. Donor killer cell Ig-like receptor B haplotypes, recipient HLA-C1, and HLA-C mismatch enhance the clinical benefit of unrelated transplantation for acute myelogenous leukemia. Journal of Immunology. 2014;**192**(10):4592-4600. DOI: 10.4049/jimmunol.1302517

Chapter 5

Laser Ablation and Immune Stimulating Interstitial Laser Thermotherapy

Cristina Pantaleone

Abstract

Based on nineteenth-century findings that showed that heat (fever) could be used to treat cancer, local hyperthermia has been developed as a tool to eradicate local tumors when surgical excision is deemed impossible. Nonetheless many cancer patients with advanced disease still lack effective treatment. During the last decades, data has emerged indicating that in situ destruction of tumors in some cases may induce tumor antigen release which can stimulate antigen-specific cellular immunity. Immune stimulating interstitial laser thermotherapy (imILT) is a method for local hyperthermia using laser light to increase tissue temperature with a specific protocol which can result in in situ vaccination. In vivo studies have shown that the method can induce an immune response that is effective against re-challenging, therefore indicating abscopal effect. Data was collected during clinical studies to assess the safety and feasibility of the method.

Keywords: local hyperthermia, laser ablation, LITT, ILT, imILT, immunooncology, laser, abscopal effect, laser ablation, local treatment

1. Introduction

The use of both light and heat in medicine has roots that reside long back in history. In ancient times, sunlight was used to treat different kinds of skin and mental diseases. These treatments mimic, amplify, and in some cases focus on natural occurring phenomena to achieve a therapeutic goal.

During the nineteenth century, it was observed that prolonged heating, as fever or locally externally induced hyperthermia, could cause cancerous formations to disappear [1–4]. Since then, many methods to treat cancer with heat were introduced, from whole body to local methods such as microwave ablation, radiofrequency ablation, and laser ablation. The main goals with innovative treatments that utilize heat are to give an alternative to patients that are not suitable for surgery and minimize the impact of the intervention on the patient. In addition, many of these methods have a lower economical impact on the treating institution budget, which enables clinics to offer treatment to a larger number of patients.

Other methods that do not make use of heat as treating source were also developed, such as cryogenic ablation that uses subfreezing temperatures to kill the tumor cells or photodynamic therapy (PDT) that uses a selective combination of light and photoactivatable drugs to induce radicals in the tumor.

 IntechOpen

Interest in focal ablation of tumors increased significantly in the last decades because of indications that local treatment may cause shrinkage of untreated, in some cases distant, tumors suggesting the involvement of the immune system in the process [5–7]. The so-called abscopal effect evoked by local treatments could be used to treat patients that lack effective treatments to date. Immune stimulating interstitial laser thermotherapy is an innovative hyperthermia treatment that uses a specifically tailored treatment protocol based on lower temperature heating for a prolonged period of time and designed to maximize the probability of triggering the immune system response to the treated tumor type. The medical device system uses laser as heat source; the same system is also used for interstitial laser ablation to burn tumorous and non-tumorous formation when imaging is challenging given its natural MR compatibility.

2. Laser-induced hyperthermia

Laser-based hyperthermia, known as laser thermotherapy or laser ablation, is a focal hyperthermia technique that uses laser light as heat source. Its minimally invasive version for treatment of tumors located deeper in the body is called interstitial laser thermotherapy (LITT or ILT). The main goal in oncological treatments is to achieve tumor destruction without damaging tissue and structures surrounding the neoplastic lesion to be treated. Different factors concur to the tissue destruction, among these direct cell death and coagulation.

During laser-induced thermotherapy, light causes damage in tissue due to absorption of light and through heat conduction into the tissue of the absorbed energy. Laser thermotherapy therefore produces a lesion that is larger than the volume where light is absorbed due to this heat conduction.

These two phenomena, direct light absorption and heat conduction, determine the modality and the parameters to be used to control the tumor heating and are dependent on the characteristics of the tissue to be treated.

2.1 Direct tissue absorption

The penetration depth, which is defined as the distance at which the light is attenuated to $1/e$ (37% of original intensity), can be used to describe the volume in which the main part of the laser energy is absorbed in tissue, i.e., where direct absorption is the dominant factor. Penetration depth can also be used to determine whether the possibility for carbonization during ablation is affected by, for example, the choice of the wavelength. Low penetration depth indicates a higher power density in tissue and thereby a higher risk of carbonization. Therefore it is an important factor to be taken into consideration both when designing the optical fibers to deliver the light and when deciding on suitable treatment parameters.

Penetration depth depends on the tissue type since the optical properties are dependent on tissue composition and structure. For a generic tissue composition, the effective attenuation coefficient and the penetration depth can be calculated as follows:

$$\mu_{eff} = \sqrt{3\mu_a\left(\mu_a + \mu_s(1 - g)\right)} \tag{1}$$

$$\delta_{eff} = 1/\mu_{eff} \tag{2}$$

Values for μ_a, μ_s, and g, in different tissue types, are available in textbooks dealing with optical properties in tissue, e.g., [8].

The absorption, μ_a, of a specific tissue depends on the tissue composition. Each component has a specific absorption spectrum. Biological tissue has a relatively low absorption in the interval 600–1200 nm. This is due to the fact that the absorption spectrum of the main component of tissues, water, has a minimum in this region. Other tissue components, especially blood, must also be considered. In **Figure 1**, only the major absorbers for the specific wavelength in use are shown.

The scattering, μ_s, depends on the tissue structure, for example, on the cell size and shape, and how they are arranged in the tissue. Light scattering in tissue has two contributions, Rayleigh and Mie scattering; the latter is usually predominant due to the scattering of particle size. The scattering is inversely proportional to the wavelength: as the wavelength increases, the scattering coefficient diminishes. As the two wavelengths considered are spectrally close, the scattering coefficients are similar. The scattering spectrum for a generic soft tissue is shown in **Figure 2** and was calculated according to [9]:

$$\mu_s = \frac{a'}{(1-g)}\left(f_{Ray}\left(\frac{\lambda}{500\,[nm]}\right)^{-4} + (1-f_{Ray})\left(\frac{\lambda}{500\,[nm]}\right)^{-b_{Mie}}\right) \qquad (3)$$

The equation takes into consideration different scattering contributions mainly due to the different sizes of the scattering centers.

All the parameters are tissue dependent. The values for a generic soft tissue in **Table 1** were used in **Figure 2**.

2.2 Heat conduction in biological tissue

The energy deposited in tissue causes an increase in temperature in the portion of tissue where laser light is absorbed. Naturally, the difference in heat evens out over time. The heat is removed from the volume where absorption of light occurs by active or passive cooling. Active cooling is achieved through blood perfusion, which varies during time according to response of the tissue to heat and is dependent on the perfusion rate and therefore on the tissue type. Passive cooling is due to heat

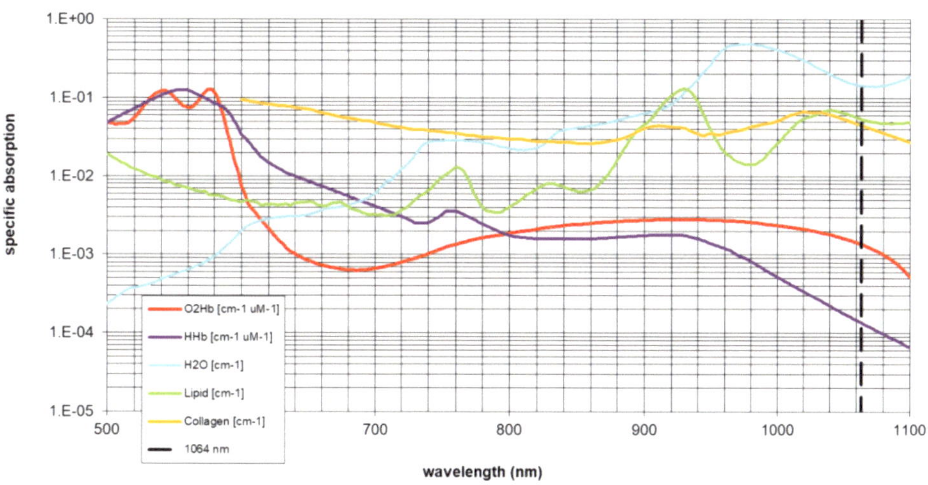

Figure 1.
Absorption spectra of tissue components in the window 500–1100 nm. Dotted line at 1064 nm.

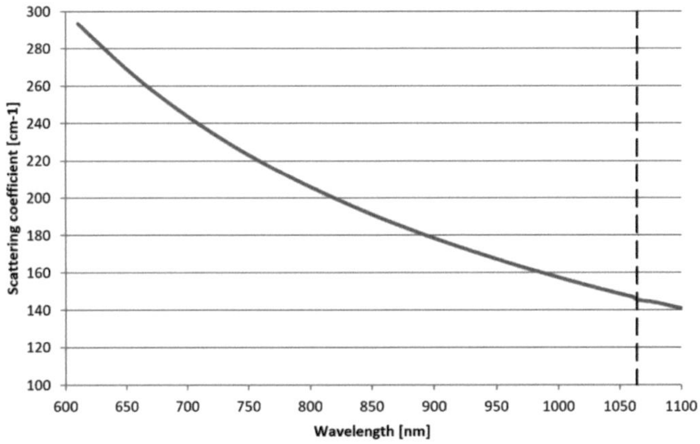

Figure 2.
Scattering coefficient for a generic soft tissue in the window 500–1100 nm, data from literature. Dotted line at 1064 nm.

g	0.95
a′ [cm^{-1}]	19.1
f_{Ray}	0.153
b_{Mie}	1.091

Table 1.
Scattering parameters for a generic tissue [9].

conduction and is described by the second law of thermodynamics which asserts that heat flows spontaneously from hot to cold bodies, in this case from the heated portion of tissue to the portion of tissue at body temperature.

If the delivered energy is high enough, the heat conduction concurs to the progression of the damage since heat conduction can cause tissue temperatures to rise well above the threshold for permanent damage. The threshold for permanent tissue damage is discussed in the following paragraphs.

Pennes' equation models heat distribution in the tissue:

$$\rho c \frac{\partial T}{\partial t} + \nabla(-k\nabla T) = \rho_b c_b \omega_b (T_b - T) + Q_{met} + Q_{ext} \quad (4)$$

The equation describes the heat flow in the tissue as the combination of (passive) heat conduction, (active) heat transport due to blood perfusion and dependent on the temperature difference, metabolic heat source which is the heat produced by the tissue itself, and the external heat source, in this case the laser energy [10–12].

2.3 Laser-induced tissue effects

Effects on biological tissues induced by lasers can vary in nature and can be classified in several groups among which are photochemical damage, when light triggers a chemical reaction in the tissue, and thermal effects, when heat is the cause of the outcome. Photochemical damage includes radical formation and tissue inflammation, while examples of thermal damage are protein denaturation and burning. The type of damage triggered depends mainly on the characteristics of the light beam (wavelength, power, pulse properties, exposure time, spot size) and if the beam is collimated, i.e., laser source.

Thermal effects are caused when the temperature in the tissue is locally increased over the physiological temperature; the threshold is generally set to 40°C. Conditional to the specific tissue properties, beam characteristics and exposure times, the tissue can undergo hyperthermia (<60°C), coagulation, vaporization, carbonization, or pyrolysis. Hyperthermia can be reversible or irreversible depending on the combination of temperature reached and exposure time. Local ablation techniques, such as microwave, radiofrequency, or laser ablation, aim at achieving a temperature of at least 60°C in the whole treated volume, therefore inducing cell death by coagulation; vaporization and carbonization may occur.

3. Laser ablation and immune stimulating interstitial laser thermotherapy (imILT)

Classic laser ablation is used to treat solid tumor masses in a variety of organs and aims at heating the whole tumor volume at a temperature of at least 60°C in order to coagulate the tissue in the area to be treated. In this way, near to instant cell death is achieved. An optical fiber is placed in the center of the region of interest, and light is delivered for a period of time of 1–10 minutes depending on the volume to ablate and the device used. The treatment can be repeated directly after to achieve larger coagulation volume either inserting the fiber in a new position or utilizing the so-called pull-back technique, meaning performing a new ablation along the insertion track by pulling the fiber back.

Immune stimulating interstitial laser thermotherapy (imILT) is a local ablation method that works at non-coagulating temperatures at the tumor border. The technique consists in creating a temperature gradient in the tumor that results in a heating to 46°C at the tumor border or some millimeters outside it. The temperature is then kept for a prolonged period of approximately 30 minutes to achieve an immunogenic cell death (ICD) at the tumor border, visible only 48–72 hours after treatment, which activates an immune response [13, 14]. An example of ablation achieved performing an imILT treatment is shown in **Figure 3**. The biological process is not fully understood to date, but the hypothesis is that imILT creates inflammation in the tumor. Damage-associated molecular pattern (DAMP) signal is created, and antigens, which are not coagulated due to the low temperatures, are released [7, 15–17]. The antigens are picked up by antigen-presenting cells (APCs) that in turn trigger an immune response [18–21].

The method can in principle be used to treat all types of solid tumors, but some types will be more responsive than others depending on the tumor biology, which is true for immunotherapies in general. Some results from proof-of-concept preclinical and clinical studies are presented in this chapter.

3.1 Technical solutions for interstitial laser thermotherapy

The CE-marked and FDA-approved TRANBERG® Thermal Therapy System for imILT consists of three main parts: a laser generator, a laser applicator, and a thermometry system. The laser generator is a diode-based system that emits light at a wavelength of 1064 nm and with a maximum accessible power of 25 W continuous wave. The unit has a built-in temperature feedback system that is able to measure the temperature in the tissue by means of a minimally invasive temperature probe and to drive the laser emission in order to maintain a stable temperature, set by the user between 43 and 50°C, for a treatment time of up to 30 minutes. The laser

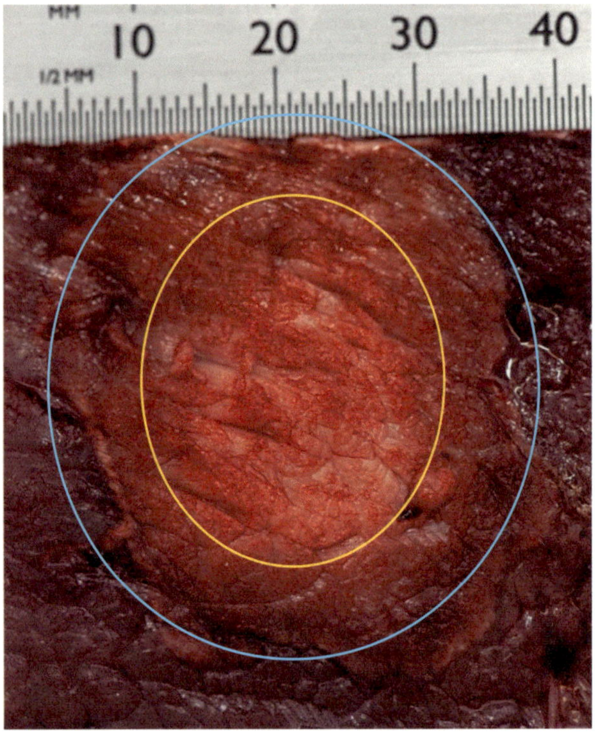

Figure 3.
Effect of imILT treatment on porcine healthy skeletal muscle tissue. Coagulation is achieved within the yellow circle, and immunogenic cell death (ICD) is achieved along the ablation border, between the yellow and the blue line.

applicator consists of a non-cooled optical fiber and an introducer to enable insertion of the fiber in the tissue. The non-cooled optical fiber is available in different tip designs tailored to the ablation volume and shape to be achieved and the tissue to be treated.

All the procedures are performed under image guidance, using MRI, ultrasound, computed tomography (CT), or a combination of the previous depending on the availability of these techniques at the clinic. While it is only possible to perform imILT treatments using ultrasound or CT guidance due to limitations in the temperature probe design, the design of the laser applicator allows laser ablation procedure to be performed with MRI guidance, for example, when performing a focused laser ablation (FLA) for the treatment of early prostate cancer or benign prostatic hyperplasia (BPH).

3.2 In vivo studies on abscopal effect of imILT

Extensive preclinical studies were performed to prove the immune stimulating effects of imILT. One specific study aimed at comparing the immunologic memory evoked by imILT if compared to resection [22].

Research was conducted on 280 rats divided in four groups: (1) rats with tumor implanted in the liver that were treated with imILT, (2) rats with tumors implanted in the liver that were treated with surgical resection, (3) rats without tumor that were treated with imILT ablating normal liver tissue (sham imILT), and (4) rats without tumors that were treated with resection of a part of a healthy liver (sham resection).

Rats in groups 1 and 2 were implanted with adenocarcinoma and treated after 6–8 days. A second challenging tumor of the same kind was implanted in another lobe 2, 5, or 10 weeks later, and the animals were followed for up to 48 days after rechallenge unless they showed signs of inactivity or distress earlier. Vital tumor at sacrifice was evaluated together with other immune system markers. Group 1, tumor treated with imILT, showed a distinct behavior if compared with the other three groups. In groups 2, 3, and 4, the challenging tumor, second implanted, displayed a growth so substantial that none of the rats survived for 48 days. On the contrary, rats in group 1 showed eradication of the challenging tumor at day 48. The extent of the tumor burden for the four groups is represented in **Figure 4**. These findings, combined with results from immunology markers from blood tests, indicate that imILT invokes a strong immune response and an immunologic memory against the treated cancer.

3.3 Clinical results

A number of pre-marketing clinical studies on imILT were performed at Lund University Hospital, Lund, Sweden, where the method was developed for the first time. These studies demonstrated the recruitment of immunocompetent cells in breast cancer patients which indicate a favorable antitumor activity [23–27].

More recently, initial findings from the clinical study program designed to evaluate the safety and the usability of the method performed using the TRANBERG®|Thermal Therapy System (Clinical Laserthermia Systems, AB, Sweden) were published [28]. A variety of solid tumors are included in the study program; the data was reported after 12 patients were treated, out of which 4 were female and 8 were male. Indications treated were breast cancer (n = 1), breast cancer metastasis (n = 1), colon cancer metastasis (n = 2), malignant melanoma metastasis (n = 2), pancreatic carcinoma (n = 1), and primary pancreatic carcinoma (n = 5); the latter two were treated in open surgery, while the other percutaneously. All the treatments were performed using CT or ultrasound guidance. All patients included in the study underwent numerous previous treatments due to comorbidity.

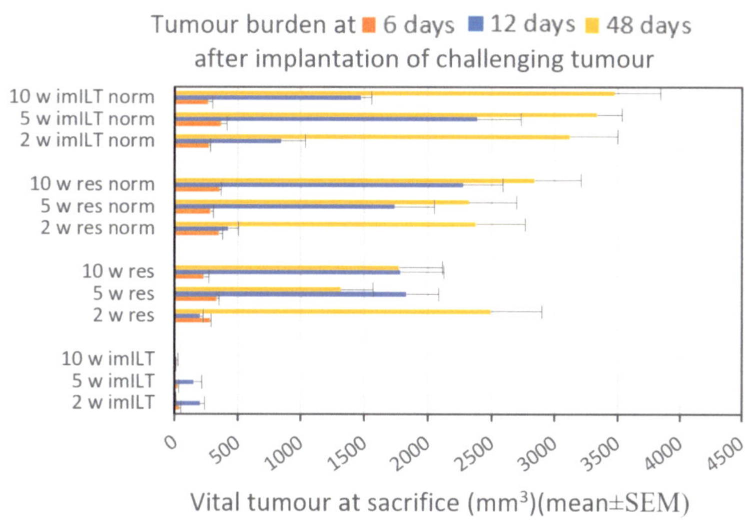

Figure 4.
Tumor burden after implantation of challenging tumor. Only rats having been treated with imILT of primary tumor survived for 48 days after implantation of challenging tumor. All other rats in the 48-day study group had to be euthanized within 10–30 days after the tumor challenge due to extensive tumor. Image: Mats Ekelund.

Immunotherapy was delivered on two malignant melanoma patients before imILT treatment but not during the study period.

One serious adverse event was reported out of nine patients within the sponsor initiated clinical study; the frequency of serious adverse events is in line with previous data on other local ablative techniques, including laser ablation [29, 30], indicating that the procedure can be safely performed.

Usability results vary among the different study clinics. Preliminary indications suggest that insertion and placement of the instrumentation within the volume to be treated are the main challenge, while sterile access, removal from the tissue, and handling of disposable are perceived as less complicated. Handling of the laser unit needs further investigation as the data is spread [28].

The safety studies were not designed to collect statistically significant efficacy results. Each study included different indications to gather safety data and input to future efficacy studies as extensive as possible leading to a low number of patients per indication, and therefore no indication-based data was published. Future ongoing publications will include indicative efficacy and quality-of-life results from these studies.

3.3.1 Case report

This case is a 53-year-old patient with pancreatic cancer diagnosed about 2 years before and treated with first-line chemotherapy, FOLFIRINOX 16 cycles, for tumor reduction. Disease progression was registered after 12 cycles. Due to intolerable toxicity, the treatment regimen was changed to second- and third-line chemotherapies, gemcitabine and protein-bound paclitaxel 16 cycles, after which partial response was achieved. At the time of the first imILT treatment 2 years after the diagnosis, the patient presented with pancreatic carcinoma and three liver metastases (stage IV). PET-CT showed a hypermetabolic focus around the biliary stent, but no clearly visible tumor in the pancreas, and three metastases in the liver (segments VI, V/VI, and V/peri-gallbladder area).

The first treatment was performed on a 19 mm liver metastasis in segment VI that was metabolically active; see **Figure 5**. The intervention was performed percutaneously under CT guidance, and a first treatment was performed by placing the tip of the radial laser applicator in the metastasis—see **Figure 6**—and a temperature

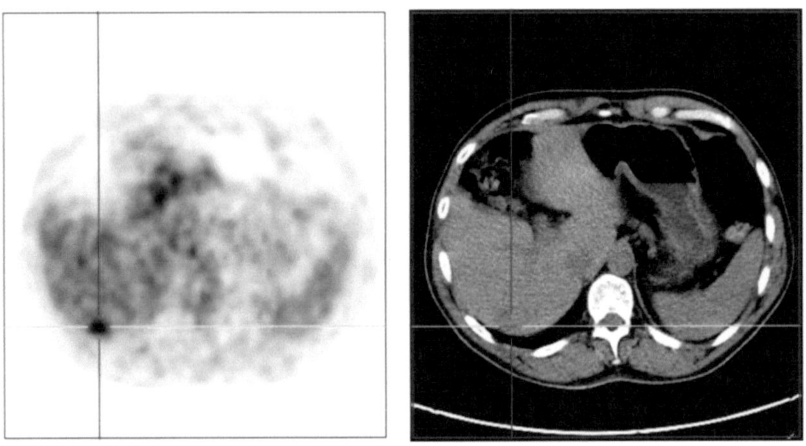

Figure 5.
PET-CT (left) and CT (right) scans showing the position of the treated metastasis during the first treatment session [31].

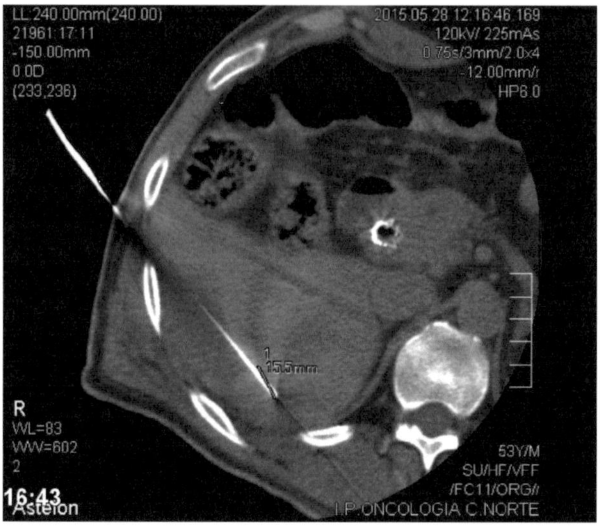

Figure 6.
Laser applicator positioning visualized using CT scan while placing the instrumentation for the first treatment [31].

needle at a distance of approximately 10 mm. The temperature needle was used to regulate the laser emission based on the measured temperature and achieve ICD in a region of the lesion that presented as metabolically active from the PET scan. A temperature of 44–45°C was kept during a period of 30 minutes according to the imILT protocol. A second overlapping ablation was performed after repositioning the laser applicator to necrotize the whole volume of the metastasis. Track ablation was performed to minimize risk for track seeding of tumor cells along the insertion track. A post-procedure CT scan was performed to ensure the ablation of the entire tumor, which was achieved as shown in **Figure 7** (black arrow). The patient suffered slight pain and rise in temperature (38°C) posttreatment, but no other

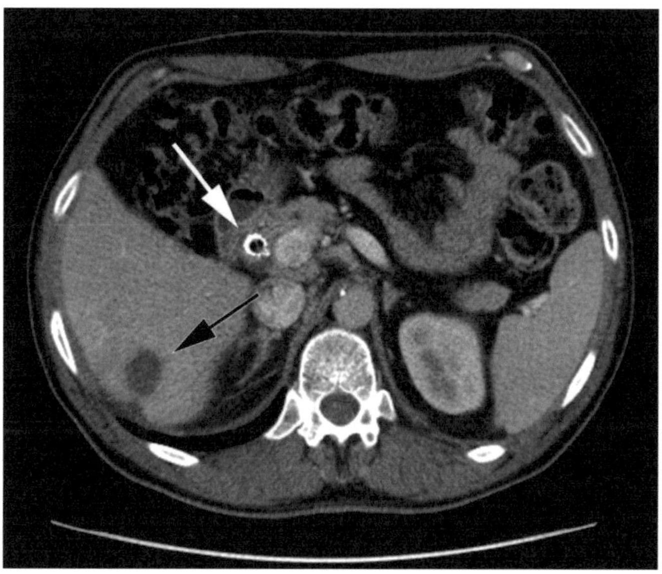

Figure 7.
Posttreatment CT that shows the ablation cavity (black arrow) and the biliary stent (white arrow). First treatment session [31].

discomfort was registered; the patient was discharged after 3 days. No complications were reported during the first 3 months following therapy [31].

Partial response in liver metastasis and total response in pancreas primary tumor were registered 21 months later. However, 3 months later disease progression was noticed, and the patient was treated with imILT for a second time 24 months after the initial treatment. The targeted metastasis was a 35 × 50 mm liver metastasis evaluated at ultrasound at the time of the treatment. The metastasis was treated performing one imILT treatment combined with an overlapping LITT treatment of about 5 minutes to necrotize the whole metastatic mass; the imILT treatment was achieved positioning the radial laser applicator off center within the tumor and the temperature probe at a distance of approximately 11 mm from the applicator. The temperature measured by the probe was kept at 43–45°C for 20 minutes.

Lastly, a third imILT treatment was performed after 40 months from the first treatment because of new disease progression. A new 20 mm liver metastasis was treated using a diffuser laser applicator combined with an introducer with built-in temperature sensors, which resulted in only one puncture. The laser applicator was inserted in the center of the metastasis, and the sensors were positioned 25 mm from the applicator tip to achieve a lesion of 25–30 mm in diameter. To date, 4 months after the last treatment, no complications connected to the laser treatment have been reported [32].

4. Conclusion

Local ablation of tumors is receiving increasing attention for the treatment of metastatic disease because of observed effects on distant tumorous masses suggesting the involvement of the immune system following local therapy.

One technique for local tumor eradication is laser ablation which kills the tumor mass by heating the tissue through direct light absorption and heat transfer resulting in tissue coagulation. imILT is an interstitial laser ablation method tailored to evoke an immune response against the treated tumor. The technique utilizes a laser applicator to deliver energy in the form of laser light to the tissue; the energy delivered to the tissue is precisely controlled based on the temperature measured by a sensor inserted in the tissue at the periphery of the tumor to obtain a lower temperature ablation that aims at maximizing the immune cell death (ICD) volume of the ablation.

Preclinical results indicate that imILT invokes an immune response against the treated tumor, if compared with resection in a rat tumor model. Clinical studies suggest that the procedure can be safely performed since the frequency of the adverse events is in line with previous data on other local ablation techniques. The case of a pancreatic cancer patient treated with imILT was presented.

Acknowledgements

This publication was founded and made possible by Clinical Laserthermia Systems AB, Lund, Sweden.

Conflict of interest

Cristina Pantaleone is the Technical Manager of Product Development at Clinical Laserthermia Systems, AB.

Thanks

I would like to thank Belarmino Gonçalves for the pictures relative to the case report and Karin Peterson, Gunilla Savring, Emily Emilsson Rossander, Maria Luisa Verteramo, and Dennis Laks for review and support.

Nomenclature

μ_a	absorption coefficient
μ_s	scattering coefficient
g	anisotropy factor
a'	scaling factor that equals the reduced scattering coefficient at 500 nm
f_{Ray}	fraction of Rayleigh scattering
b_{Mie}	scattering power (Mie scattering)
ρ	tissue density
ρ_b	blood density
k	tissue thermal conductivity
c	tissue heat capacity
c_b	blood heat capacity
ω_b	blood perfusion rate
T_b-T	difference between the heated tissue and the blood or the surrounding tissue
Q_{met}	metabolic heat
Q_{ext}	external heat sources
BPH	benign prostate hyperplasia
DAMP	damage associated molecular pattern
CT	computed tomography
ICD	immunogenic cell death
ILT	interstitial laser thermotherapy
imILT	immune stimulating interstitial laser thermotherapy
LITT	laser-induced thermotherapy
PDT	photodynamic therapy

Author details

Cristina Pantaleone
Technical Manager Product Development at Clinical Laserthermia Systems AB, Lund, Sweden

*Address all correspondence to: cristina.pantaleone@clinicallaser.com

IntechOpen

© 2019 The Author(s). Licensee IntechOpen. This chapter is distributed under the terms of the Creative Commons Attribution License (http://creativecommons.org/licenses/by/3.0), which permits unrestricted use, distribution, and reproduction in any medium, provided the original work is properly cited.

References

[1] Busch W. Uber den Einfluss, welchen heftigere Erysipl zuweilen auf organisierte neubildungen ausuben. Vol. 23. Rhein. Westph: Verhanl. Naturh. Preuss; 1866. pp. 28-30

[2] Coley WB. The treatment of malignant tumors by repeat inoculations of erysipelas: With a report of ten original class. The American Journal of the Medical Sciences. 1893;**105**:487-511

[3] Coley WB. The therapeutic value of the mixed toxins of the streptococcus of erysipelas and bacillus prodigiosus in the treatment of inoperable malignant tumors. American Journal of Surgery. 1896;**112**:251-280

[4] Westermark N. Uber die Behandlung des ulcerierenden Cervix-carcinoms mittels konstanter Wärme. Vol. 22. Zbl Gynäk. 1898. pp. 1335-1339

[5] Isbert C, Boerner A, Ritz JP, Schuppan D, Buh HJ, Germer CT. In-situ ablation of experimental liver metastases delays and reduces residual intrahepatic tumour growth and peritoneal tumour spread compared with hepatic resection. The British Journal of Surgery. 2002;**89**:1252-1259

[6] Yantorno C, Soanes WA, Gonder MJ, Shulman S. Studies in cryoimmunology. I. the production of antibodies to urogenital tissue in consequence of freezing treatment. Immunology. 1967;**12**:395-410

[7] den Brok MHMGM, Sutmuller RPM, van der Voort R, Bennink EJ, Figdor CG, Ruers TJM, et al. In situ tumor ablation creates an antigen source for the generation of antitumor immunity. Cancer Research. 2004;**64**:4024-4029

[8] Roggan A, Dörschel K, Minet O, Wolff D, GSL M. The optical properties of biological tissue in the near infrared wavelength range - review and measurements. SPIE Press. 1995;**PM25**:10-44

[9] Jacques SSL. Optical properties of biological tissues: A review. Physics in Medicine and Biology. 2013;**58**:R37-R61

[10] Nguyen TH, Park S, Hlaing KK, Kang HW. Temperature feedback-controlled photothermal treatment with diffusing applicator: Theoretical and experimental evaluations. The Journal of the Optical Society of America. 2016;**7**(5)

[11] Lakhssassi A, Kengne E, Semmaoui H. Modifed Pennes' equation modelling bio-heat transfer in living tissues: Analytical and numerical analysis. Natural Science. 2010;**2**(12):1375-1385

[12] Saccomandi P, Schena E, Silvestri S. Design of fiber optic applicators for laser interstitial thermotherapy: Theoretical evaluation of thermal outcomes. In Proceedings: IEEE Engineering in Medicine and Biology Society. 2013;**2013**:3733-3736. DOI: 10.1109/EMBC.2013.6610355

[13] Galluzzi L, Buqué A, Kepp O, Zitvogel L, Kroemer G. Immunological effects of conventional chemotherapy and targeted anticancer agents. Cancer Cell Review. 2015;**28**(6):690-714

[14] Cook AM, Lesterhuis WJ, Nowak AK, Lake RA. Chemotherapy and immunotherapy: Mapping the road ahead. Current Opinion in Immunology. 2016;**39**:23-29

[15] Chu KF, Dupuy DE. Thermal ablation of tumours: Biological mechanisms and advances in therapy. Nature Reviews. 2014;**14**(3):199-208

[16] Mellman I, Coukos G, Dranoff G. Cancer immunotherapy comes of age. Nature. 2011;**480**(7378):480-489

[17] Zerbini A, Pilli M, Penna A, Pelosi G, Schianchi C, Molinari A, et al. Radiofrequency thermal ablation of hepatocellular carcinoma liver nodules can activate and enhance tumor-specific T-cell responses. Cancer Research. 2006;**66**(2):1139-1146

[18] Gallucci S, Lolkema M, Matzinger P. Natural adjuvants: Endogenous activators of dendritic cells. Nature Medicine. 1999;**5**:1249-1255

[19] Sauter B, Albert ML, Francisco L, Larsson M, Somersan S, Bhardwaj N, et al. Consequences of cell death: Exposure to necrotic tumor cells, but not primary tissue cells or apoptotic cells, induces the maturation of immunostimulatory dendritic cells. Journal of Experimental Medicine. 2000;**191**(3):423-434

[20] Sturesson C, Ivarsson K, Andersson-Engels S, Tranberg KG. Changes in local hepatic blood perfusion during interstitial laser-induced thermotherapy of normal rat liver measured by interstitial laser doppler flowmetry. Lasers in Medical Science. 1999;**14**:143-149

[21] Sturesson C, Ivarsson K, Stenram U, Andersson-Engels S, Tranberg KG. Interstitial laser thermotherapy of a rat liver tumour: Effect of hepatic inflow occlusion. Lasers in Surgery and Medicine. 2011;**43**:29-35

[22] Ivarsson K, Myllymäki L, Jansner K, Stenram U, Tranberg KG. Resistance to tumour challenge after tumour laser thermotherapy is associated with a cellular immune response. British Journal of Cancer. 2005;**93**:435-440

[23] Tranberg KG, Möller PH, Hannesson P, Stenram U. Interstitial laser treatment of malignant tumours: Initial experience. European Journal of Surgical Oncology. 1996;**22**:47-54

[24] Tranberg KG, Ivarsson K, Willner J, Håkansson L, Stenram U. Induction of a distant anti-tumour effect by interstitial laser thermotherapy (imILT) in a patient with malignant melanoma. In: 2nd International Conference on Tumor Microenvironment: Progression, Therapy and Prevention; Baden, Austria. 2002. p. 49

[25] Haraldsdottir KH, Ivarsson K, Götberg S, Ingvar C, Stenram U, Tranberg KG. Interstitial laser thermotherapy (ILT) of breast cancer. European Journal of Surgical Oncology. 2008;**34**:739-745

[26] Haraldsdottir KH, Ivarsson K, Jansner K, Stenram U, Tranberg KG. Changes in immunocompetent cells after interstitial laser thermotherapy of breast cancer. Cancer Immunology, Immunotherapy. 2011;**60**:847-856

[27] Haraldsdottir KH, Ingvar C, Stenram U, Tranberg KG. Long-term follow-up after interstitial laser thermotherapy of breast cancer. Anticancer Research. 2015;**35**:6147-6152

[28] Axelsson J, Pantaleone C, Åstrom S. Initial findings of immunostimulating interstitial laser thermotherapy of solid tumours. Journal for Clinical Studies. 2017;**9**(4):28-31

[29] Vogl TJ, Straub R, Eichler K, Woitaschek D, Mack M. Malignant liver tumors treated with MR imaging-guided laser-induced thermotherapy: Experience with complications in 899 patients (2,520 lesions). Radiology. 2002;**225**:367-377

[30] Paiella S, Salvia R, Girelli R, Frigerio I, Giardino A, D'Onofrio M, et al. Role of local ablative techniques radiofrequency ablation and irreversible electroporation in the treatment of pancreatic cancer. Updates in Surgery. 2016:2-6

[31] Axelsson J, Pantaleone C, Dymling S, Bergenfeldt M, Sousa MJ, Machado M, et al. Successful Treatment of Pancreatic Cancer Liver Metastasis Using Immunostimulating Interstitial Laser Thermotherapy (imILT). Available from: https://clinicallaser.se/wp-content/uploads/2017/05/Poster_CLS_Porto_May_2017.pdf

[32] Gonçalves B, Sousa MJ, Machado M, Santos L. P-66 Abscopal effect of immunostimulating laser thermotherapy on liver metastasis in pancreatic cancer: A case report and study protocol for a randomised controlled trial. In: European Conference on Interventional Oncology; 8-11 April 2019; Amsterdam, The Netherlands. 2019

Chapter 6

Surgical Treatment of Benign Spinal Cord Tumors

Xiaoming Qi, Frank Y. Shan, Dongxia Feng and Jason H. Huang

Abstract

Benign spinal cord tumors (SCTs) are uncommon neoplasms that can arise within or adjacent to the spinal cord. Depending on their anatomical location, benign SCTs can be categorized as intramedullary, intradural-extramedullary, and extradural. The three most common benign SCTs are meningioma, nerve sheath tumors, and ependymoma. Both meningioma and nerve sheath tumors develop in the intradural-extramedullary compartment, while ependymoma occurs in the intramedullary space. Spinal meningiomas derive from arachnoidal cells and most commonly occur within the thoracic segment of the spine. Nerve sheath tumors, including schwannomas and neurofibromas, are closely associated with spinal nerves. Half of the spinal cord ependymomas arise in the lumbosacral segment or the filum terminale. Surgical treatment of large or symptomatic benign SCTs concentrates on total or subtotal resection of the tumors, which should be cautiously individualized based on the tumor location and histopathology. A curable complete resection should be achieved if possible while preserving the nervous function of the spinal cord and minimizing potential complications. Thoracic spinal roots may be sacrificed to acquire a total resection, yet cervical and lumbar nerve roots should be preserved prudently. Due to the vulnerable and complex anatomic nature of the spinal cord, maximal resection of the tumors can be achieved with the aid of appropriate intraoperative neural monitoring and meanwhile preserve nervous function.

Keywords: benign spinal cord tumors, surgical treatment, pathology of benign spinal cord tumors, CSF leakage

1. Benign spinal cord tumors

Spinal cord tumors are abnormal mass of tissue that could occur within or adjacent to the spinal cord. They can be benign or malignant. Benign spinal cord tumors are usually rare primary tumors originating in the spinal or spinal cord. Based on their location, they can be categorized as intramedullary, intradural-extramedullary, and extradural (**Figure 1**).

Intramedullary tumors arise inside the spinal cord itself, typically derived from glial or ependymal cells. Astrocytoma and ependymoma are the two most common types, and they usually occur in the cervical segments. Intradural-extramedullary spinal cord tumors arise within the dura but outside of the spinal cord. The most common types are meningiomas, nerve sheath tumors including schwannomas and

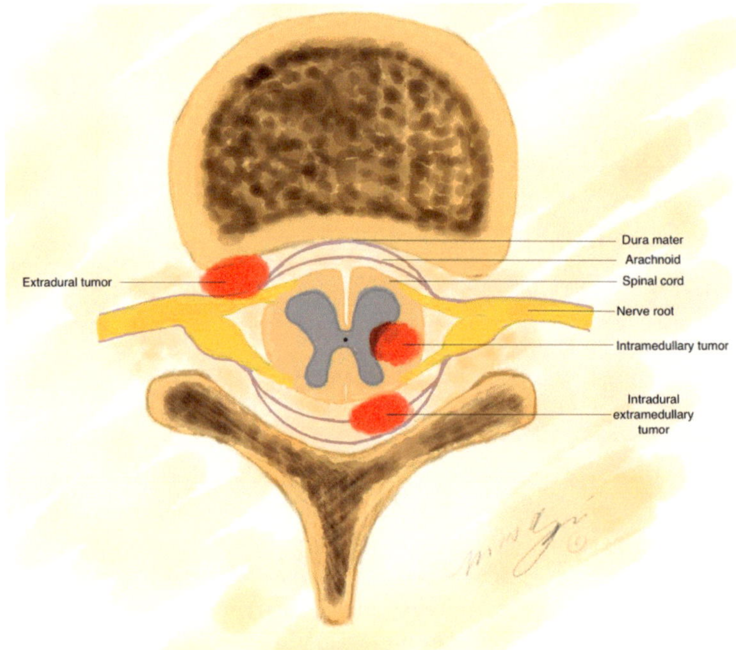

Figure 1.
Illustration of spinal cord tumor locations: intramedullary, intradural-extramedullary, and extradural.

neurofibromas, and myxopapillary ependymomas that occur on the filum terminalis and the conus medullaris. Extradural spinal cord tumors are mostly metastatic and malignant, which is not covered here.

2. Symptoms

Early symptoms of spinal cord neoplasms are often nonspecific. Gradually worsening back pain is the initial feature of spinal cord neoplastic disease in about 90% of adult patients. Spinal cord compression can have a subtle presentation. Pain often precedes other symptoms associated with spinal cord compression and causes nocturnal awakening. Discomfort may be radicular, localized to the back, or both. Patients often describe this pain as a gnawing and unremitting. Radicular pain suggests nerve root impingement and may provide an indication of the location of the tumor. Neurologic dysfunction distal to the lesion is due to interruption of ascending and descending spinal cord pathways. The most common sequelae are sensory dysesthesias and muscular weakness, especially of the iliopsoas musculature. Once symptoms other than pain appear, they may progress rapidly. Tumors intrinsic or extrinsic to the spinal cord can cause symptoms through disruption of normal neural elements and pathways, producing both local and distal effects. Sensory or motor symptoms that may be referred to the cord include limb paresthesia and weakness. Paraplegia and bowel or bladder disturbances (e.g., constipation, urinary hesitancy, retention, incontinence) are usually late findings except in conus medullaris syndrome, in which sphincter dysfunction and saddle anesthesia may emerge early in the course. Although neurologic manifestations may begin unilaterally, they can progress to involve both sides of the spinal cord and thereby produce bilateral symptoms and signs.

3. Physical examination

Findings on physical examination could define a probable site of tumor, document preoperative neurologic deficits, and determine progressive neurologic deterioration. They usually correspond to the location of the tumor, degree of cord impingement, and duration. Early in the course of spinal cord compression, spasticity, hyperreflexia, and loss of pinprick, temperature, position, and vibratory sensation may occur, while the Babinski may be absent. Tenderness over the affected spinal region can present. Late in the course of spinal cord compression, weakness, clear sensory loss, bilateral Babinski signs, and decreased anal sphincter tone, hyperreflexia and Babinski can be present. Lax rectal sphincter tone is a late sign of spinal cord dysfunction. Lhermitte's sign suggests irritation of the meningeal irritation. Brown-Sequard syndrome is caused by lateral spinal cord compression. Cauda equina syndrome and conus medullaris syndrome can be present as a result of compression of the spinal cord and nerve roots arising from L1–L5 levels.

4. Pathology

4.1 Intramedullary tumors

The majority of intramedullary primary spinal cord tumors are gliomas. Due to the relative paucity of glial tissue in the spinal cord, spinal cord gliomas are rare compared to their cerebral counterparts. The major types of spinal glial tumors are ependymomas and astrocytomas.

4.2 Ependymomas

Ependymomas are intramedullary tumors that may be located anywhere along the spinal cord. Over 50% occurs in the filum terminale; the other 50% can occur anywhere in the cervical or thoracic spinal cord [1]. In the World Health Organization (WHO) classification of brain tumors, ependymal tumors are divided into four major groups: sub-ependymoma (WHO Grade I), myxopapillary ependymoma (WHO Grade I), ependymoma (WHO Grade II), and anaplastic ependymoma (WHO Grade III).

4.3 Ependymoma

Ependymomas are more common in adults, with a peak age at presentation between 30 and 40 years. Histologically, they can be categorized to papillary, cellular, epithelial, or mixed. The cellular subtype is most common. Clinically, patients often have localized pain for months to years prior to developing other symptoms leading to diagnosis. Physical exam findings include lower extremity spasticity, loss of pain and temperature sensation, lower extremity and truncal sensory diminution to light touch and vibration, as well as gait ataxia. Ependymomas tend to arise centrally within the cord and expand symmetrically as they grow. Cystic degeneration occurs in about 46% of the cases [2, 3]. They are usually encapsulated and minimally vascular. These lesions generally enhance intensely on MRI. Optimal management consists of gross total resection. Although these are infiltrative tumors, a total or near-total resection can frequently be achieved without causing further neurologic deficits.

4.4 Myxopapillary ependymoma

Myxopapillary ependymomas are biologically and morphologically distinct from other ependymomas (**Figures 2** and **3**). These tumors most commonly arise in the conus medullaris and the filum terminale. At this anatomic location, ganglioglioma and lipoma are the second and third most commonly seen tumors separately following myxopapillary ependymoma. Myxopapillary ependymomas are WHO Grade I and usually solitary. They are papillary with microcystic vacuoles. Myxopapillary ependymomas are slow-growing glial tumors, sometimes with an indolent course for long periods of time. They typically are found in young male, with a median age at diagnosis from 35 to 37 years, and a male to female ratio ranging from 1.4 to 2.5 to 1 [4, 5]. Myxopapillary ependymomas generally present with low back pain, with or without radicular features. The vast majority of these tumors are located in the lumbosacral or thoracolumbar spine. Initial management of these tumors consists of laminectomy with attempted surgical resection. These tumors oftentimes can be totally resected, and many patients are cured following gross total resection. Subtotal resection deems necessary in particular with unencapsulated tumors. As postoperative radiotherapy tends to improve local control and prolong the recurrence-free interval, it may be considered in patients who have undergone subtotal resection or biopsy of a myxopapillary ependymoma. However, radiotherapy is still controversial since its effect on overall survival is unclear.

4.5 Astrocytomas

Astrocytomas occur throughout the spinal cord with the thoracic segment being the most common site. Approximately 50% of spinal cord astrocytomas is pilocytic, and 50% is infiltrative astrocytomas. Pilocytic astrocytomas are well circumscribed and low grade with nonaggressive clinical behavior. On MRI these tumors enhance intensely with gadolinium. Low-grade astrocytomas are shown as hypointense to

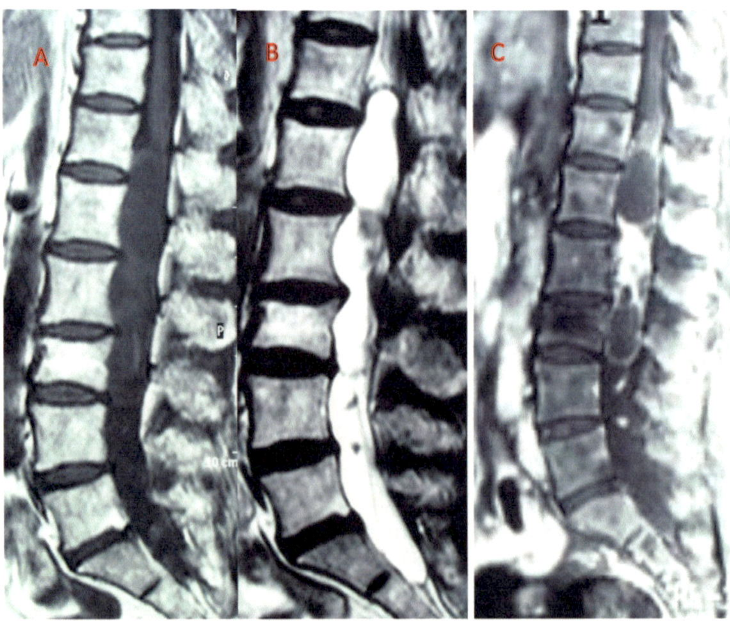

Figure 2.
Encapsulated myxopapillary ependymoma: (A) T1WI shows isointense mass, (B) T2WI shows slightly hyperintense mass with capsule, and (C) T1 with contrast shows enhancement of the mass.

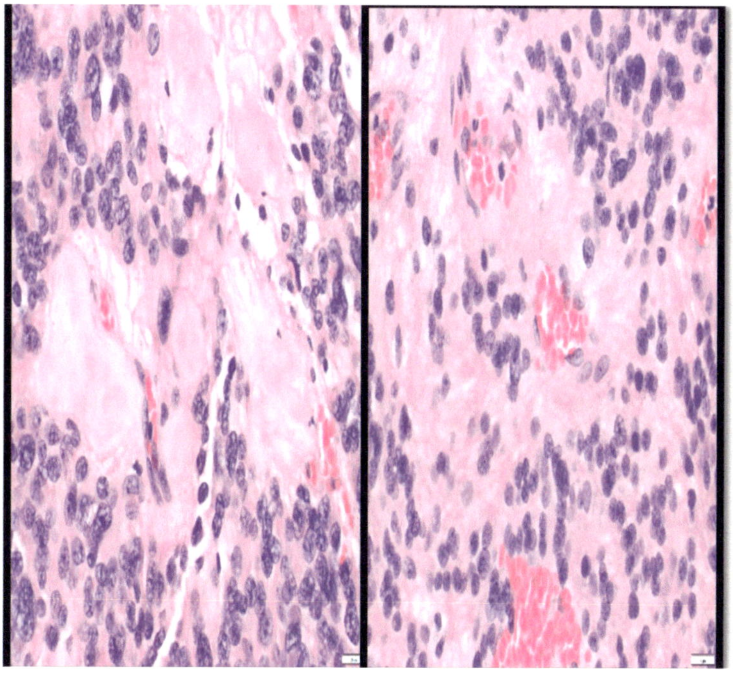

Figure 3.
Focal hyalinized vessels (left) and perivascular pseudorosettes (right) are characteristic histological features of WHO Grade I myxopapillary ependymoma.

isointense signal on T1-weighted images and hyperintense signal on T2-weighted images [6]. Diffuse fibrillary astrocytomas of the spinal cord usually appear as nonencapsulated lesions that enhance minimally or heterogeneously on MRI with gadolinium. Peak diagnosis ranging from the third to the fifth decade, with a median age 35 years. Male to female ratios are about 1.5 to 1. The most important factor associated with a better prognosis is low tumor grade (WHO Grade I). Other factors associated with a better prognosis include tumor location other than the cervical region, limited extent of tumor involvement along the spinal cord, and longer (>180 days) duration of symptoms. Postoperative radiotherapy does not affect outcomes in patients with pilocytic astrocytomas. The initial step in the management of a patient with a symptomatic or enlarging presumed primary intramedullary spinal cord tumor is a surgical procedure for tissue diagnosis and resection to the maximum extent possible. Pilocytic astrocytomas can often be completely or near-completely resected without causing further neurologic deficits. Diffuse fibrillary astrocytomas are more infiltrative, and meaningful resection is often precluded by the lack of clear tissue planes and high risk of neurologic morbidity, in which case an internal debulking procedure would be performed.

5. Intradural-extramedullary tumors

Both meningiomas and nerve sheath tumors (schwannomas and neurofibromas) can develop in the intradural-extramedullary spinal compartment.

5.1 Meningioma

Meningiomas can arise from arachnoidal cap cells anywhere along the neuraxis. Spinal meningiomas most commonly arise within the thoracic spine. Over three fourths occur in women. The tumors are frequently adherent to the spinal dura, requiring dural resection for complete removal. The tumors can be intradural, extradural, and a mixture of intradural and extradural. Psammomatous meningiomas are the most common histological subtypes of spinal meningioma (**Figure 4**). Spinal meningiomas are typically slowly growing, invasive lesions and may remodel or erode bone. Pathologically, spinal meningiomas demonstrate the same features seen with intracranial lesions. Calcifications may be suggestive of the histologic diagnosis of meningioma. Local or radicular pain is the most common symptom associated with spinal meningiomas, followed by motor deficits and sensory symptoms. On MRI, meningiomas are iso- to hypointense on T1 and slightly hyperintense on T2, with a strong and homogeneous enhancement with gadolinium (**Figure 5**). The usual treatment for spinal meningiomas is resection, and complete resection can often be achieved. The dural origin is generally cauterized and occasionally resected. Thoracic spinal roots may be sacrificed as necessary to achieve a complete resection; cervical and lumbar nerve roots are preserved whenever possible. Recurrence rate with complete excision is 7% [7]. Subtotally resected lesions are generally followed expectantly for regrowth. Symptomatic recurrences are generally treated with further surgery.

5.2 Nerve sheath tumors

Nerve sheath tumors constitute about 25% of tumors arising from the dorsal sensory root near the edge of its exit from the spinal canal in the intradural-extramedullary space. Majority of nerve sheath tumors are schwannomas (**Figure 6A**), and most of the remainder are neurofibromas. Nuclear palisading (Verocay bodies) is a typical feature in schwannomas, with spindle cells arranged in short, intersecting fascicles. Neurofibromas grow as fusiform expansions of the involved nerve. They are less compact and less cellular than schwannomas. Spindle-shaped tumor cells with a wavier or buckled nuclear profile are typical to neurofibromas. Schwannomas and neurofibromas typically are slow growing. Patients generally present with local pain initially, which typically worsens at night or in the morning and resolves during the day. Neurologic deficits develop late in the course of the disease when they fill a significant volume of the spinal canal. As the tumor grows, it extends to the epidural space through the narrowest portion of the course of the nerve root, forming a "dumbbell-shaped" tumor (**Figure 6B**), which is rather radiographically typical. Small, asymptomatic tumors are best observed with serial imaging before committing to definitive surgical therapy. Large or symptomatic tumors are best treated with surgeries. The goal of the surgery is to achieve gross total resection of the benign

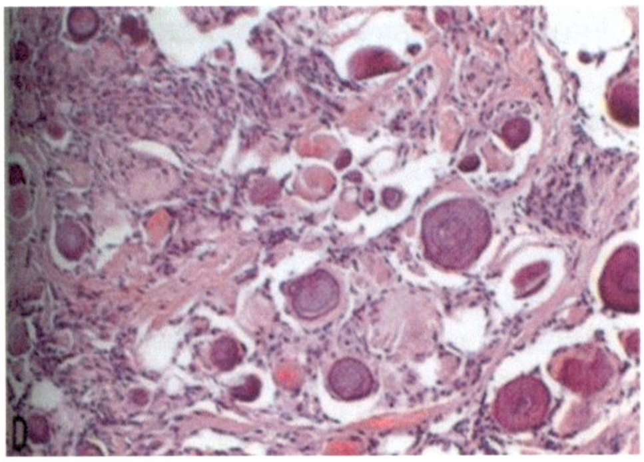

Figure 4.
WHO Grade I psammomatous meningioma, a predominant subtype of meningioma in the spinal region.

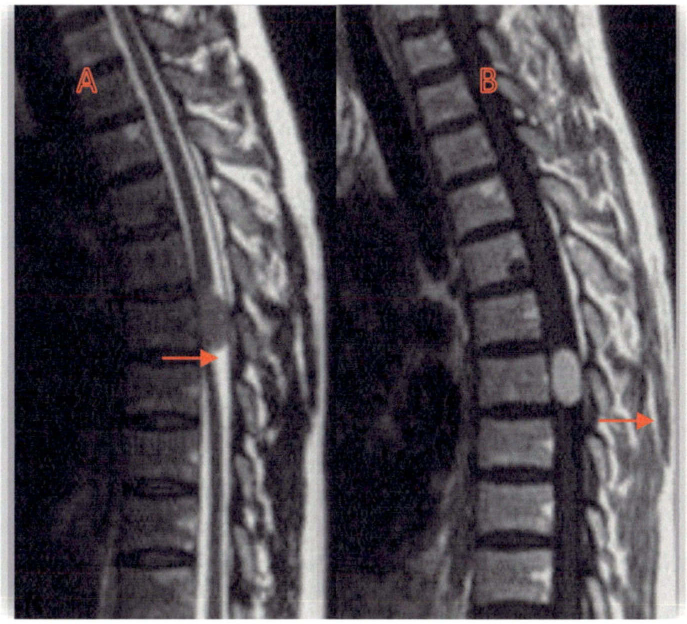

Figure 5.
(A) T2WI, a round slightly hyperintense mass is seen in the intradural space. (B) MRI contrast image shows homogeneous enhancement.

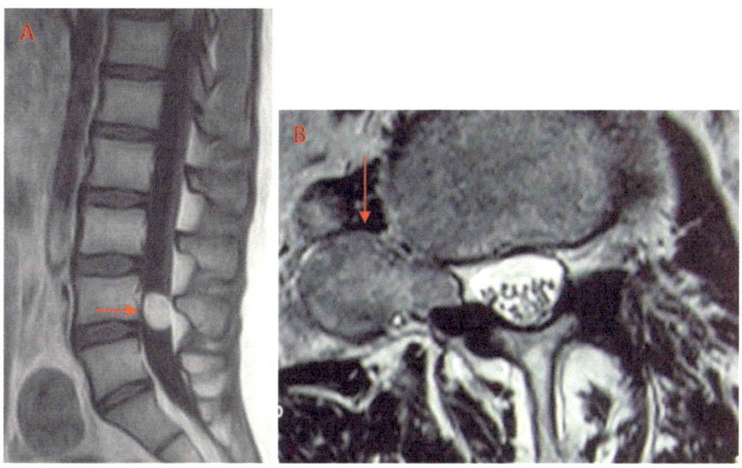

Figure 6.
(A) T1 with contrast: Schwannoma shows enhancement and (B) T2WI shows a "dumbbell-shaped" schwannoma.

tumors, yet a subtotal resection should be obtained to spare neurological function impairment as most of the tumors are benign and slow growing.

6. Surgical treatment

6.1 Surgical anatomy

The adult spine consists of 33 individual vertebrae, which are divided into the cervical, thoracic, lumbar, sacral, and coccygeal vertebrae. The vertebrae are joined by cartilaginous interbody joints, synovial facet joints, spinal ligaments, and overlying muscles and fasciae. The vertebral foramina constitute the vertebral canal, which contains the spinal cord, nerve roots, meninges, and vasculatures. Adjacent vertebrae form the intervertebral foramina laterally, where the spinal nerves and vessels go through. The posterior portion of the vertebra is called the vertebral arch, which consists of a pair of pedicles and a pair of laminae supporting articular processes, transverse processes, and the spinous process. Reconstruction of the vertebral arch is critical in a surgical treatment of spinal tumors via a posterior surgical approach (**Figure 7**).

The spinal cord runs within the superior two thirds of the vertebral canal from the medulla oblongata to the conus medullaris. The anterior median fissure extends along the whole ventral surface and runs deeper caudally. The posterior median sulcus is shallower, from which a posterior median septum penetrates more than halfway in to the spinal cord. The septum diminishes caudally as the canal becomes more dorsally placed. Lateral to each side of the posterior median sulcus lies the posterolateral sulcus, along which the dorsal roots of spinal nerves enter the cord. Between the posterolateral sulcus and anterior median fissure is the anterolateral funiculus, where the ventral spinal rootlets pass through.

The paired dorsal and ventral roots of the spinal nerves are continuous with the spinal cord. They unite in or close to their correspondent intervertebral foramina to form the spinal nerves. There are 31 pairs of spinal nerves branching off the spinal cord. The section of spinal cord associated with the emergence of a pair of nerves is named a spinal segment.

The conus medullaris is the tapered, lower end of the spinal cord near L1 or L2 vertebra. The upper conus medullaris is usually not well defined. The level at which the spinal cord ends variates in population. The vertebra column elongates more rapidly than the spinal cord during development, hence the discrepancy between the anatomical level of spinal cord segments and their corresponding vertebrae. The spinal nerves continue to branch out after the conus medullaris, forming the cauda equina, which is gathered round the filum terminale. The pia mater surrounding

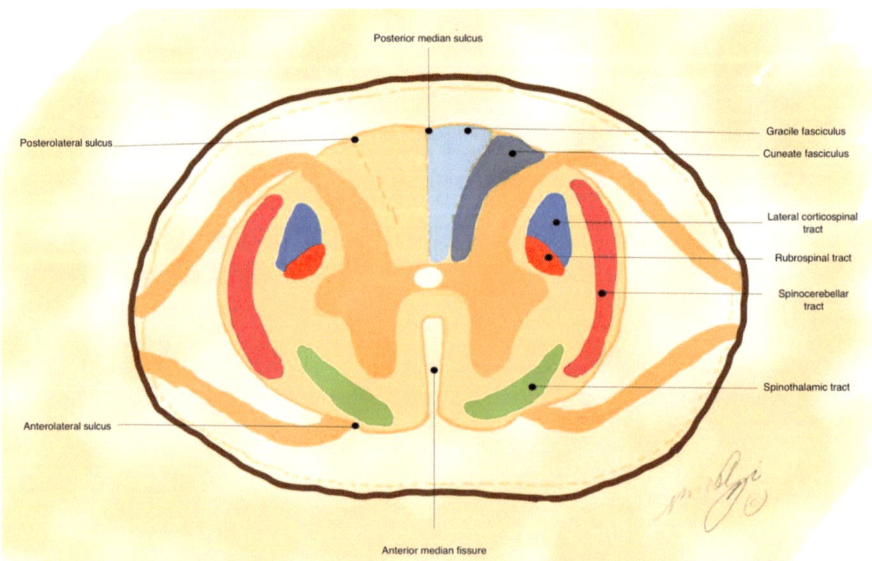

Figure 7.
Illustration of a cross-section anatomy of the spinal cord showing deep anterior median fissure, shallow posterior median sulcus, and shallow grooves of anterolateral or posterolateral sulcus.

the spinal cord projects directly downward, forming the filum terminale. The filum terminale, descending from the apex of the conus medullaris, is continued within extensions of the dural and arachnoid meninges and reaches the caudal border of the second sacral vertebra, stabilizing the entire spinal cord.

The spinal cord is covered by the meninges. The outermost membrane is the spinal dura mater which forms a tube. The spinal cord is directly covered by the thin, translucent membrane of the pia mater, which itself comprises an inner membranous layer, the intima pia, and a more superficial epipial layer. The intima pia, adherent to the underlying nervous tissue, follows its contours closely. The epipial layer is formed by a mesh network of collagenous fiber bundles continuous with the arachnoid trabeculae, as what we call an intermediate leptomeningeal. The blood vessels of the spinal cord lie within this epipial layer. This intermediate leptomeningeal layer is closely applied to the innermost aspect of the arachnoid membrane; it reflects to form the dorsal septum and arborizes over the dorsal surface of the spinal cord, resulting in the formation of the epipial layer. The anterior spinal arteries and veins are arborized over by a dense epipial layer. The spinal cord is attached to the dura mater by a series of lateral, flattened bands of epipial tissue known as the dentate ligaments. The spinal dura mater extends around the spinal roots and nerves as they pass through the vertebral canal and the intervertebral foramina. These prolongations of spinal dura mater are called spinal nerve sheaths or root sheaths. The arachnoid within the sheaths does not extend as far as their dural coverings. Limited prolongation of the arachnoid demonstrates the nerve sleeves.

7. Surgical treatment

The posterior midline approach is most frequently used to remove tumors. Even ventrally located lesions can be safely resected via posterior approach. Dentate ligament resection allows for general mobilization of the spinal cord. Posterior roots can be sacrificed from C2 to C4 and throughout the thoracic region. Lower cervical and lumbosacral posterior roots should be preserved whenever possible. If it becomes necessary to sacrifice the sensory nerve root, it should be resected proximally to the ganglion to minimize postoperative neuralgia. Intracapsular decompression could be required for larger tumors. In a dumbbell-shaped tumor, the intradural portion should be resected first to minimize spinal cord manipulation during the excision of the extradural component. The dura must be closed in a watertight fashion. In cases where a meningioma required resection of dura, a dural graft should be utilized for a watertight closure of the dura to prevent CSF leakage.

7.1 Intramedullary tumors

Surgery is the treatment of choice or the only effective treatment for intramedullary spinal cord tumors. Most patients experience some loss of posterior column function following surgery due to the performance of the myelotomy through the posterior median septum. Due to the indolent feature of benign intramedullary tumors, it is important to optimize both the timing and the performance of surgery in these patients. The goals of surgical treatment are to preserve neurologic function and to maximize surgical removal. These goals are generally compatible, but the preservation of neurologic function should always come first. For patients with an incidental finding of asymptomatic intramedullary tumor, serial imaging and clinical follow-up are recommended. Once symptoms commence, then surgery is offered, before the onset of any substantial neurologic deficit, because surgery is usually not effective in reversing neurologic deficits.

Cysts are frequently found at both ends of a tumor, which serve as landmarks in the dissection. The true tumor-cord interface needs to be carefully exposed, especially in possible cases of benign encapsulated tumors, with minimal damage to the spinal cord parenchyma. It is crucial to identify tumor-cord interface. When a clear tumor-cord interface is difficult or the intraoperative appearance of the tumor suggests an anaplastic nature, further tumor removal is not warranted. Majority of intramedullary ependymomas can be totally resected with preservation of neurologic function, as they usually have a clear plane of dissection. Resection of low-grade astrocytomas should be continued until the interface with the spinal cord is recognized. The interface is not always distinguishable. Surgical resection of more malignant astrocytomas is still controversial, as improvement of neurologic function is still unclear. Hemangioblastomas are well circumscribed and encapsulated neoplasms, so gross total resection can be achieved in nearly all cases. However, they are highly vascular, and vascular supply should be totally interrupted before the removal of the tumor. In general, assessment of the tumor-spinal cord interface under the operating microscope is the most important factor in determining the specific surgical objective for each patient with a benign intramedullary lesion, irrespective of tumor histology.

7.2 Extramedullary tumors

The goal of management for patients with extramedullary spinal cord tumors is either long-term tumor control or cure with preservation of neurologic function. Surgery is clearly indicated in patients with symptomatic tumors particularly those with large tumors producing significant compression of the spinal cord or cauda equina. For patients with smaller tumors or those with minimal subjective symptoms, it may be considered to follow them both over time. For small and asymptomatic tumors, regular radiographic surveillance can also be recommended. However, midline filum/cauda equina tumors are usually ependymomas in nature, which can disseminate through CSF; therefore, an early total resection of these lesions is recommended. The vast majority of intradural-extramedullary tumors can be safely accessed and removed through a standard posterior laminectomy. Even most ventrally located tumors can be accessed posteriorly because lateral spinal cord displacement or rotation enables a safe corridor to debulk and remove most ventrally located tumors. However, pure ventral lesions may require a more lateral or, rarely, an anterior approach. Intraoperative ultrasound can be used to identify the location of the tumor levels. Dumbbell tumors with epidural extension into the neural foramen usually require a unilateral facetectomy to allow access to foramina, followed by instrumented fusion extending one level above and below the facetectomy. Whenever possible, it is preferable to remove the tumor through a single operative exposure to reduce morbidity and preserve surgical options. Debulking is recommended when the tumor is large. As the tumor is mobilized, the nerve stimulator is used to identify motor roots. Once the root or rootlet of origin has been identified, it is sectioned both proximally and distally, and the tumor is removed. If the tumor extends into the extradural space, motor stimulation is essential to determine whether there is motor root involvement. If there is no motor root stimulation, the entire root can be sacrificed. However, a functional motor root involved by tumor should be spared to avoid a significant postoperative neurologic deficit, even though this produces a subtotal resection.

8. Technical advances and adjunctive options

Ultrasonic surgical aspiration: this device consists of a hollow tube that vibrates at high frequencies and physically emulsifies the tumor while irrigating and aspirating the field. It improves the debulking of spinal tumors. When placing the aspirator tip in contact with the tumor, the surgeon can achieve a relatively atraumatic resection of the tumor, without manipulation of the adjacent spinal cord. Additionally, the ultrasonic aspirator allows preservation of blood flow in adjacent tissue.

8.1 Intraoperative ultrasonography

With an ultrasonic transmitter placed over the spinal cord, intraoperative ultrasonography can help identify the location of the tumor, existence of intramedullary cysts, and the relationship between the spinal cord and the surrounding structures. Prior to dural opening, bony exposure can be adjusted, which could reduce the possibility of further bone removal after dural opening and minimize the risk of direct injury of the exposed neural structures. The integration of intraoperative ultrasonography and microscope allows for a better visualization of the surgical field and to facilitate tumor resection. It can also assist with identifying any residual tumor tissue after resection. A color flow Doppler ultrasound can be utilized for a vascular tumor like hemangioblastoma or in a case where major vasculature structure has been involved. By allowing the evaluation of the anatomy underneath surgical field surface, intraoperative ultrasonography can help in refining the surgical strategy.

8.2 Intraoperative neurophysiological monitoring

Intraoperative neurophysiological monitoring has gained popularity with surgeons when it comes to a surgical resection of intramedullary tumor. Somatosensory evoked potential (SSEP) and transcranial motor evoked potential (MEP) are the most commonly used techniques which continuously monitor sensory and motor potentials individually during surgery for intramedullary tumors. With transcranial MEP, motor pathways are stimulated centrally, and responses can be recorded directly from needle electrodes placed in the extremities' muscles. Myogenic MEP waveforms recorded from muscles can be categorized into three patterns: polyphasic, biphasic, and absent. An electrophysiologist will view and record waveforms and their changes and report any possible adverse reactions to the descending motor pathways related to the surgery. Intraoperative neurophysiological monitoring is not absolutely reliable, as a change in potential may not present until up to 1 minute after the occurrence of the injury [8]. Due to the proximity of the corticospinal and spinothalamic tracts, as well as the dorsal columns, intraoperative injury to the motor pathways can be reflected in changes in sensory evoked potentials. MEP monitoring can be used to avoid excessive spinal cord manipulation and improve the surgical technique during resection of the tumor. Amplitude changes in MEP have been examined to be strongly correlated with postoperative neurologic function [9, 10].

9. Outcome of treatment

9.1 Intramedullary tumors

With aggressive surgical resection as the treatment of choice, postoperative neurologic outcome is closely related to the patient's preoperative neurologic status. In general, better postoperative neurologic outcome occurs with lesser preoperative neurologic deficits [11]. It has been argued that postoperative deterioration of neurologic function, regardless of being transient or permanent, is attributed to direct surgical insult to either the spinal parenchyma or the spinal cord circulation. When a posterior median sulcus approach is used, patients may present posterior column dysfunction early after surgery, including abnormalities of discriminative touch sensation, proprioception, or gait [12]. These symptoms may or may not be permanent. Neuropathic pain syndrome can present after surgery when syringomyelia is associated with the lesion.

When low-grade astrocytoma is associated with a cyst, a clear interface can be identified between the tumor and the spinal cord; a gross total resection of the lesion is optimal. This will halt the clinical and radiological progression of the tumor for many months. Due to the infiltrative nature of high-grade astrocytoma, radical resection of the lesion is not feasible without damaging the normal spinal cord tissue. Progression of low-grade astrocytoma into high-grade tumor can occur, which then further affects the outcome. For patients with ependymomas, long-term survival is expected, especially as total resection of the tumor is widely adopted. In comparison to astrocytoma, the outcomes of ependymomas do not appear to be related to histologic grades of the tumor. Although rare, CSF dissemination of ependymoma does occur.

9.2 Extramedullary tumors

Regardless of tumor histology, location, and extent of lamina resection, the surgical outcomes of extramedullary tumors are optimal in general [13, 14]. However, an early surgical intervention is recommended for symptomatic lesions, as it is associated with a greater postoperative improvement [13]. Neurologic complications are uncommon, and even if they do occur, improvement could be expected in majority of the cases. Improvement of initial neurologic deficits can be expected for months and up to a year after tumor resection. Provided that a gross resection has been obtained, recurrence rarely occurs [15]. In the case where recurrence does occur, reoperation is usually not required instantly and largely contingent on the patient's neurologic status, age, and tumor growth rate captured with a series of radiologic images.

10. Complications

10.1 CSF leakage

The incidence of CSF leakage remains high after spinal cord tumor surgeries involving opening of the dura mater. It is more commonly seen in the upper thoracic region. Radiation therapy prior to the surgery is a risk factor for patient to develop a CSF leak. Improper treatment of CSF leakage can potentially give rise to other complications including CSF fistula, meningitis, abscess, and even neurological deficits [16].

Management of CSF leakage entails two aspects based on CSF dynamics [17]: to prevent CSF leak with direct watertight closure of the dura mater and to retard CSF leak by reducing the subarachnoid CSF pressure and/or increasing the epidural space pressure. Prevention is of great importance in managing CSF leakage complication. A watertight closure of the dura mater is crucial, and a direct suture with adjuvant dural closure material has gained popularity among spinal surgeons owing to its high successful rate in watertight closure [18, 19]. At times the involved dura has been inevitably excised, and this renders a primary closure impossible. In this case, an augmented closure with the aid of an adipose tissue, muscle tissue, or fascial graft would be indicated. The graft would be layered over the defect of dura mater, and prolonged bed rest with a wound drainage would be warranted to avoid a CSF leakage [20–22]. In the event of CSF leakage development, techniques reducing the subarachnoid fluid pressure would be exploited. This includes inhibiting the formation of CSF with medications such as acetazolamide, adjusting patient's position, and CSF shunting with a lumbar drain placement [16, 23]. These approaches have been proven effective, although complications do occur pertinent to the treatment [24, 25].

CSF leakage is a vexing problem and usually requires prolonged postoperative treatment. Should CSF leakage persist, surgical exploration of proper dura closure may deem necessary and should not be delayed.

10.2 Postoperative instability

Due to the generally optimal neurological outcome of extramedullary spinal tumors, a rising attention has been turned to the long-term outcome after tumor resection involving a spine procedure. Postoperative iatrogenic instability has been recognized throughout different spine segments, including cervical kyphosis after laminectomies, thoracic instability after laminoforaminotomy-facet resections, and spondylolisthesis after lumbar laminectomies [26, 27]. This has been attributed to the alteration in spine biomechanics as a result of extensive laminectomies with or without facetectomies [28]. Postoperative instability is associated with preoperative instability, extent of facetectomy, level of spine segments involved, and disruption of ligamentous structures. Stabilization is warranted in patient demonstrating preexisting spine instability. An increasing number of levels involved entail more disruptions of structural components during the procedure, which results in a higher risk of postoperative instability [29]. A biomechanical model study has shown that removing the medial one third to one half of the facet joint as well as the posterior ligaments destabilizes the spine by significantly increasing spinal flexion by nearly 12° [30]. Instrumented fusion that extends one level above and below the facetectomy is usually performed. If instability happens, it should be identified early, and a stabilization procedure should be performed to arrest the progression. In patients who are treated with cervical region tumors involving extensive laminectomies, stabilization is routinely applied. Post-laminectomy kyphosis is exceedingly difficult to treat; thus, surgical stabilization is imperative to preempt this [31].

Minimal invasive procedures have prevailed among spinal surgeons; however, their indications are largely contingent on each individual case, and their efficacies in preventing instability have yet to be determined.

11. Summary

Substantial advancement of neuroradiology and its wide adoption in clinical settings have improved the recognition of spinal cord tumors. Many lesions have now been identified on MRI before they become symptomatic clinically. Early recognition has offered physicians the advantage of managing and treating these tumors in the early course of the disease. General refinement of surgical techniques and adjunctive technologies has undeniably improved the outcome of the disease while minimizing neurologic deficits.

Author details

Xiaoming Qi, Frank Y. Shan*, Dongxia Feng and Jason H. Huang
Department of Neurosurgery, Baylor Scott and White Medical Center, College of Medicine, Texas A&M University, Temple, Texas, USA

*Address all correspondence to: yshan918@gmail.com

IntechOpen

© 2019 The Author(s). Licensee IntechOpen. This chapter is distributed under the terms of the Creative Commons Attribution License (http://creativecommons.org/licenses/by/3.0), which permits unrestricted use, distribution, and reproduction in any medium, provided the original work is properly cited.

References

[1] Waldron JN, Laperriere NJ, Jaakkimainen L, et al. Spinal cord ependymomas: A retrospective analysis of 59 cases. International Journal of Radiation Oncology, Biology, Physics. 1993;**27**:223

[2] McCormick PC, Torres R, Post KD, Stein BM. Intramedullary ependymoma of the spinal cord. Journal of Neurosurgery. 1990;**72**:523

[3] Kumar R, Reeddy SJ, Wani AA, Pal L. Primary spinal primitive neuroectodermal tumor: Case series and review of the literature. Pediatric Neurosurgery. 2007;**43**:1-6

[4] Pica A, Miller R, Villà S, et al. The results of surgery, with or without radiotherapy, for primary spinal myxopapillary ependymoma: A retrospective study from the rare cancer network. International Journal of Radiation Oncology, Biology, Physics. 2009;**74**:1114

[5] Weber DC, Wang Y, Miller R, et al. Long-term outcome of patients with spinal myxopapillary ependymoma: Treatment results from the MD Anderson Cancer Center and institutions from the Rare Cancer Network. Neuro-Oncology. 2015;**17**:588

[6] Van Goethem JW, van den Hauwe L, Ozsarlak O, et al. Spinal tumors. European Journal of Radiology. 2004;**50**:159-176

[7] Solero CL, Fornari M, Giombini S, Lasio G, Oliveri G, Cimino C, et al. Spinal meningiomas: Review of 174 operated cases. Neurosurgery. 1989;**25**:153-160

[8] Kobayashi S, Matsuyama Y, Shinomiya K, Kawabata S, Ando M, Kanchiku T, et al. A new alarm point of transcranial electrical stimulation motor evoked potentials for intraoperative spinal cord monitoring: A prospective multicenter study from the Spinal Cord monitoring Working group of the Japanese Society for Spine Surgery and Related Research. Journal of Neurosurgery. Spine. 2014;**20**:102-107

[9] Kothbauer KF. Intraoperative neurophysiologic monitoring for intramedullary spinal-cord tumor surgery. Neurophysiologie Clinique. 2007;**37**:407-414

[10] Cheng JS, Ivan ME, Stapleton CJ, Quinones-hinojosa A, Gupta N, KI A. Intraoperative changes in transcranial motor evoked potentials and somatosensory evoked potentials predicting outcome in children with intramedullary spinal cord tumors. Journal of Neurosurgery. Pediatrics. 2014;**13**:591-599

[11] Matsuyama Y, Sakai Y, Katayama Y, Imagama S, Ito Z, Wakao N, et al. Surgical results of intramedullary spinal cord tumor with spinal cord monitoring to guide extent of resection. Journal of Neurosurgery. Spine. 2009;**10**:404-413

[12] Brotchi J. Intrinsic spinal cord tumor resection. Neurosurgery. 2002;**50**:1059-1063

[13] Byvaltsev VA, Damdinov BB, Belykh EG, Ivanova KO, Sorokovikov VA, Tsunetoshi K, et al. Neurosurgical outcomes of intradural extramedullary spinal tumors in 97 cases: Siberian Experience. No Shinkei Geka. 2017;**45**(9):781-787

[14] Bokhari I, Rehman L, Farooq G, Qureshi A. Postoperative functional outcome of intradural extramedullary spinal tumors through posterior approach. Journal of the College of Physicians and Surgeons–Pakistan. 2016;**26**(2):117-120

[15] Gilard V, Goia A, Ferracci FX, Marguet F, Magne N, Langlois O, et al. Spinal meningioma and factors predictive of post-operative deterioration. Journal of Neuro-Oncology. 2018;**140**(1):49-54

[16] Menon SK, Onyia CU. A short review on a complication of lumbar spine surgery: CSF leak. Clinical Neurology and Neurosurgery. 2015;**139**:248-251

[17] Fang Z, Tian R, Jia YT, Xu TT, Liu Y. Treatment of cerebrospinal fluid leak after spine surgery. Chinese Journal of Traumatology. 2017;**20**(2):81-83. DOI: 10.1016/j.cjtee.2016.12.002. Epub 2017 Feb 24. Review

[18] Kim KD, Wright NM. Polyethylene glycol hydrogel spinal sealant (DuraSeal Spinal Sealant) as an adjunct to sutured dural repair in the spine: Results of a prospective, multicenter randomized controlled study. Spine (Phila Pa 1976). 2011;**36**:1906-1912

[19] Wright NM, Park J, Tew JM, et al. Spinal sealant system provides better intraoperative water tight closure than standard of care during spinal surgery: A prospective, multicenter, randomized controlled study. Spine (Phila Pa 1976). 2015;**40**:505-513

[20] Turel MK, D'Souza WP, Rajshekhar V. Hemilaminectomy approach for intradural extramedullary spinal tumors: An analysis of 164 patients. Neurosurgical Focus. 2015;**39**(2):E9

[21] Arnautovic K, Arnautovic A. Extramedullary intradural spinal tumors: A review of modern diagnostic and treatment options and a report of a series. Bosnian Journal of Basic Medical Sciences. 2009;**9**(suppl 1):40-45. Review

[22] Chabok SY, Safaie M, Ashraf A, et al. Effect of fat graft on dural tear repair in lumbar spine laminectomy surgery. Neurosurgery. 2014;**24**:1-4

[23] Abrishamkar S, Khalighinejad N, Moein P. Analysing the effect of early acetazolamide administration on patients with a high risk of permanent cerebrospinal fluid leakage. Acta Medica Iranica. 2013;**51**:467-471

[24] Farhat HI, Elhammady MS, Levi AD, et al. Cervical subarachnoid catheter placement for continuous cerebrospinal fluid drainage: A safe and efficacious alternative to the classic lumbar cistern drain. Neurosurgery. 2011;**68**:52-56

[25] Açikbaş SC, Akyüz M, Kazan S, et al. Complications of closed continuous lumbar drainage of cerebrospinal fluid. Acta Neurochirurgica. 2002;**144**:475-480

[26] Bevevino AJ, Helgeson MD, Albert TJ. Iatrogenic spinal instability: Cervical and thoracic spine. Seminars in Spine Surgery. 2013;**25**:119-130

[27] Lee Y-P, Sclafani J. Lumbar iatrogenic spinal instability. Seminars in Spine Surgery. 2013;**25**:131-137

[28] Hammerberg KW. New concepts on the pathogenesis and classification of spondylolisthesis. Spine (Phila Pa 1976). 2005;**30**(suppl):S4-S11

[29] Lee KK, Teo EC, Qiu TX, Yang K. Effect of facetectomy on lumbar spinal stability under sagittal plane loadings. Spine (Phila Pa 1976). 2004;**29**:1624-1631

[30] Abumi K, Panjabi MM, Kramer KM, Duranceau J, Oxland T, Crisco JJ. Biomechanical evaluation of lumbar spinal stability after graded facetectomies. Spine (Phila Pa 1976). 1990;**15**:1142-1147

[31] Anderson DG, Silbert J, Albert TJ. Management of cervical kyphosis caused by surgery, degenerative disease, or trauma. In: Clark C, editor. The Cervical Spine. 4th ed. Philadelphia: Lippincott Williams & Wilkins; 2005. pp. 1135-1146